Everything You Need To Know About Buying Prescription Drugs
in the U.S., Canada and Mexico

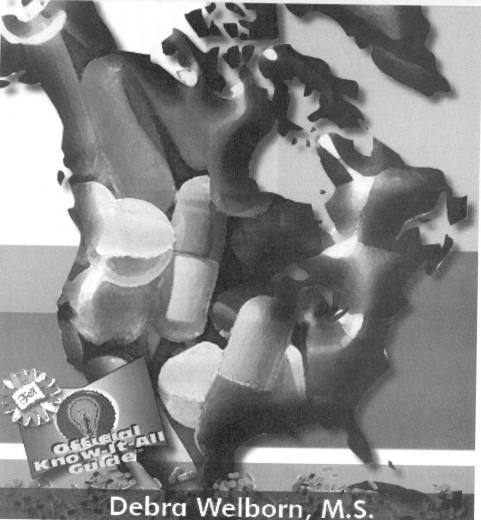

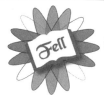

Official Know-It-All Guide™

Debra Welborn, M.S.

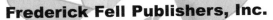

Frederick Fell Publishers, Inc.

2131 Hollywood Boulevard, Suite 305

Hollywood, Florida 33020

954-925-5242

e-mail: fellpub@aol.com

Visit our Web site at www.fellpub.com

This publication is designed to provide accurate and authoritative information in regard to the subject matter covered. *This book is not intended to replace the advice and guidance of a trained physician nor is it intended to encourage self-treatment of illness or medical disease. Although the case histories presented are true, all names of patients have been changed.*

Library of Congress Cataloging-in-Publication Data

Welborn, Debra,
 Everything You Need To Know About Buying Prescription Drugs in the U.S., Canada and Mexico *by Debra Welborn*
       p. cm.
   ISBN 0-88391-412-6 (trade pbk. : alk. paper)
   1. Medical I. General Interest.
   GV995.R55 2005
   744572--dc246
                          2005018814

Cover and Interior Design- Chris Hetzer, It's About Time Productions

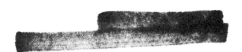

Everything You Need To Know About

Buying Prescription Drugs in the U.S., Canada and Mexico

By Debra Welborn, M.S.

For Norma St. John, my mother.

Thanks for always watching over me.

ACKNOWLEDGEMENTS

Many thanks to my son Morgan Welborn and my sister Kathy St.John, who have supported me over the past two years as I turned my passion into a reality. I owe gratitude, as well as lunch, to my many friends and colleagues for their support and encouragement. Among them are: Rosemary, Marilyn, Sara, Helen, Stella, Debbie, Jennifer, Karin, Kena, Margie and Karl. Also, many thanks to my publisher at Frederick Fell Publishers, Inc. for his belief in this project.

DISCLAIMER

Throughout this book, various brand names are used. Such trademarks are the property of their respective owners. The author's use of these trademarks should not be construed as an affiliation or sponsorship of any kind.

Every effort has been made to provide a guide for buying prescription drugs that is accurate, complete, and concise as possible. However, *everything* to do with prescription drugs is constantly changing and many facts are contradictory. The author and publisher personally do not endorse the use of any particular pharmacy, website, or store, but believe the information written this book, if made available to the public, will allow consumers to make their own informed choices. Readers should always consult their personal healthcare professional(s) concerning any questions they have about their prescription and non-prescription drug therapy. Ultimately, the decisions on what, where and when to purchase prescription drugs (from foreign internet sites or any other sources) is *entirely* up to the reader.

TABLE OF CONTENTS

FOREWARD

This is a MUST book for every household......considering that three-fourths of all Americans purchased at least one prescription drug this past year. You can go the best doctor, receive treatment in a first class hospital, but if you cannot afford your meds, take your meds the wrong way, or take meds that interact with each other in a negative way...then all the evaluation by the doctor will not translate into making you healthy. An educated consumer of health care is much more likely to use the health care system effectively. Debra Welborn does a superb job of providing a comprehensive review of essential information about meds and a clear understanding of the pricing of medications.

I am honored to have the opportunity to introduce you to this book. You can use it as a reference, or read it straight through....either way, this book is empowering. It puts you in the driver's seat and gives you the tools to make wise decisions about where to buy your medications at affordable prices. The book also gives you the big picture of the pharmaceutical industry... how a med goes from discovery to your medicine cabinet and how this process is regulated.

Neil Shulman, M.D.
Author and Associate Producer of Doc Hollywood
Associate Professor of Emory University School of Medicine
Author: Your Body's Red Light Warning Signals:
Medical Tips to Save Your Life
www.redlightwarningsignals.com and What's in a Doctor's Bag?

Introduction

Why this book?

Have you ever walked into a drugstore to purchase your prescription drugs, only to walk out feeling like you were ripped off? If you have, you are not alone. Rarely a day goes by that you don't see an article about the high cost of prescription drugs in a magazine or newspaper. Prescription drugs have become not only a monthly household expense, but in many cases, a "big ticket" item. In the U.S., the average annual cost of prescription drugs is approximately $449.00 per person.[1] However, some American families spend $3,000 or more per person per year. This amount can be more than a family's annual utility bill(s).

The costs (as well as the usage) of prescription drugs continue to rise. Prescription drug sales in 2004 increased by 8.2% to a whopping **$221 billion** in wholesale dollars[2]. Prescription drugs continue to become an increasingly larger component of medical treatment and health care costs, with spending more than tripling since 1990.

Little 'colored pills" have become the panacea for a young and healthy life. And why not? Pharmacotherapy was one of the most significant medical contributions of the 20th century and continues to play a major role in health care in the 21st century. Prescription drugs have increased longevity and have allowed Americans to have a better quality of life.

Due to the fact that prescription medications effect almost every American on a daily basis, it's important to obtain as much knowledge about taking and buying prescription drugs as possible. While there is no shortage of information about prescription drugs available to the public, it is often confusing and contradictory. Much of the information is inaccurate, and even dangerous. For the average consumer, it's almost impossible to make wise, cost-effective choices about prescription drug therapy.

Consider the following true-life examples:

50-year-old John S. takes antibiotics for frequent sore throats. If he can't purchase his prescription through his physician, he buys fish antibiotics from the pet store.

45-year-old Joan B. takes Claritin for sinusitis. Claritin is now available over the counter (OTC). Joan doesn't know whether a prescription alternative is a better choice (e.g. Claritin Rx), but in any cases, she doesn't want to purchase an OTC product if it's more expensive than her HMO copay of $10.00.

25-year-old Joshua has a receding hairline. He wants to buy Propecia over the Internet because he doesn't have insurance. Plus, he can't afford a doctor's visit for the prescription. Even if the Propecia sold over the Internet is less expensive, Joshua doubts if the drug is of the same quality as the one he usually purchases at the local drugstore for a much higher price.

2-year-old Janey has an ear infection. Her mom takes her to the Hospital Emergency Room at night and receives a prescription for a new powerful antibiotic. When she arrives at her local pharmacy, she is informed that the drug is *not* on her HMO formulary and there is no generic equivalent available for that specific drug. Now Janey has a very sick child and no antibiotic that can be covered by her HMO until the pharmacist can contact her physician and ask for a substitute drug during office hours the next day.

76-year-old Mildred K. can't afford her prescription drugs because Medicare doesn't offer a prescription drug benefit. She's now making monthly trips across the border to Canada to buy them at a 40% discount. She worries that she's breaking the law and that she'll find herself hauled off to prison in handcuffs.

Many Americans have faced challenges such as the ones listed above in their efforts to obtain affordable drug therapy. The lack of prescription drug coverage and the high cost of prescription drugs is part of the health care crisis in this country today.

Why I wanted to be the one to write this book

After working in the healthcare industry for 30 years, I found the idea of writing a book that would help people save money on prescriptions drugs to be very appealing. I've had the opportunity to work in many health-care environments and had both the satisfaction and the challenge of try-ing to make the pieces of the pharmaceutical puzzle fit together. At HMOs, I struggled to provide cost-containment strategies by negotiating discount prices and implementing formularies. (See Chapter 6). At two pharmaceutical firms, I was employed as a sales representative and while there, I engaged in all the accepted industry practices calculated to increase sales for my companies. I experienced first hand the free-mar-ket system and how it works in regards to pharmaceuticals. I realized that most Americans are unaware of what happens behind the scenes way before a patient ever steps up to the "drop off" window at his or her local pharmacy to buy a prescription drug.

My education and career experience, coupled with the real life experi-ence of being a single mother who at one time was unable to afford med-ications for her son, gives me the knowledge as well as the passion, to write this book. I wanted the opportunity to share helpful tips about com-parison-shopping for prescription drugs.

How can readers use the information in this book?

In the past, you might never have even known what questions to ask in order to shop around for prescription drug discounts. This book will give you the questions *and* the answers. It is designed to be a reference- a vital source of general information about prescription drug therapy. You will also find information regarding non-prescription drug therapy (OTCs) since many times there other options to the high-cost brand name drugs. Americans are usually very savvy consumers. They shop around for bar-gains and they know how to buy at discounts. In fact, Americans know more about shopping for everything from automobiles to avocados than they do about shopping for prescription drugs at discounted prices. Although prescription drugs should never be considered average consumable goods, the same principles that say there are price variations, fluctuations and discount strategies for all products is more analogous than one might think. This book will assist readers in their "comparison shopping" by presenting all the facts and comparisons required to do a painless yet thorough job.

How is the book organized?

This book is designed so that readers can find their particular area of interest and go directly to that information without reading all the chapters in chronological order. I recommend that you review the Table of Contents and skim through the APPENDIX to find specific areas of interest as well as pertinent price comparisons

The Book is divided into the following parts:

Part 1- Prescription Drugs 101

Part 1 provides valuable clinical information to assist readers in purchasing prescription drugs in the United States. Several chapters discuss general issues such as what exactly is a drug, what is the difference between generic and brand name drugs and when it is appropriate to purchase over-the-counter drugs. Other chapters will discuss the FDA, pharmaceutical companies, Medicare, HMOs and discount card programs.

Part II- Buying Prescription Drugs in the U.S.

Here you will find information on how to find discounts from your local drugstore as well as tips on purchasing prescription drugs from *U.S. Internet websites. Note: Buying prescription drugs in the U.S. is still the best choice.*

Part III- Buying Prescription Drugs in Canada

Part III describes the how and why of purchasing prescription drugs in Canada. NOTE: IN MOST CASES, IT IS ILLEGAL FOR U.S. CITIZENS TO PURCHASE PRESCRIPTION DRUGS FROM CANADA,

MEXICO OR ANY FOREIGN COUNTRY FOR USE HERE AT HOME. This is the true whether the drugs are purchased via a foreign Internet website or across a foreign country's land border. However, millions of Americans continue to do so. Part III will assist readers in weighing the pros and cons of this common practice. The FDA is not yet arresting busloads of senior citizens returning from Canada, but legal actions remains a constant threat to those that purchase from a foreign country. And since Americans continue this practice, knowing the consequences, is it done perhaps with the hope that we can all impact legislation and/or bring enough media attention to effect change in drug pricing schemes? Is this common practice a type of political dissent to put downward pressure on prices and to work towards the day when it won't be necessary for Americans to travel to another country in order to afford brand name prescription drugs?

Please be advised however, that this book was written to provide the reader with information about purchasing prescription drugs in Canada and <u>not</u> to condone the breaking of any laws. If the law changes to allow reimportation, the author's website will be updated to provide further cost analysis and tips in successfully navigating any new policies.

Part IV- Buying Prescription Drugs in Europe

Here, a brief chapter exists on buying prescription drugs from European countries. This is currently done via the Internet, not by purchasing from individual countries such as Israel, Germany, India, etc. As drug companies make it more difficult to obtain purchases from Canada, Europe is becoming a more popular choice.

Part V- Buying Prescription Drugs in Mexico

Part IV discusses the practice of buying prescription drugs in Mexico or from a Mexico website. THIS IS DISCUSSED IN THE BOOK BUT <u>NOT</u> RECOMMENDED. There are severe safety concerns and it's recommended that U.S. consumers <u>not</u> buy prescription drugs in Mexico, especially for serious health conditions.

Part VI- Prescription Pathways

One of the most important parts of this book is Part VI which includes "Prescription Pathways" so that readers can find the best "path" for their particular circumstances. For example, if a reader is a Medicare recipient there is a pathway for that. If a reader has no prescription drug coverage and needs to purchase brand name drugs, there is a pathway for that. Most pathways will also lead back to specific chapters for more details. There are more Prescription Pathways posted on the website at www.prescriptionpathway.com. There is also a chapter to give readers an "Rx tune-up" and a chapter on the future of prescription drugs.

APPENDIX

In the APPENDIX, you will find many useful tools including price comparisons for the 100+ most prescribed drugs Price comparisons are included for generics and brands purchased from a mass merchandising retailer, a local pharmacy, and both U.S. and Canadian Internet pharmacies. I urge you to use APPENDIX A to comparison shop for all the prescription drugs you and your family members are purchasing. You will then find a cost savings worksheet in the APPENDIX D to calculate potential yearly savings. In addition, you will find a medication record/card that slips inside your checkbook, which lists the 3 vital questions you need to ask your physician, pharmacist and/or other healthcare practitioner when receiving a new prescription. On the reverse side of the card you will find a place to record a medication list. This card can be used during your physician office visits to stimulate a discussion with your health care practitioner(s) regarding reasons for the prescribed drug, possible contraindications and drug interactions, etc. In the last APPENDIX, readers will find information about the author's web site: www.prescriptionpathway.com. With the listed user name and password, readers will have free access to updates on prescription drugs, legislation, Medicare updates, counterfeit news, costs, etc. Also, readers will be eligible to receive a free newsletter from the site.

A note about Using Personal Stories called "It Could Happen To You"

Throughout the book you will find personal stories called "It Could Happen to You". These are real life experiences that all readers can relate to and will serve to demonstrate that most people share the same struggles in understanding the prescription drug "maze".

Use the "Tips"

Most chapters include "TIPS" on the first page. Readers should use these tips to find cost saving and/or safety information.

Important Message

Each individual's clinicians/pharmacists *are and always will be* the best source for *prescribing information* for prescription drugs. A person's health care professional(s) knows more about a patient's individual health conditions than anyone else. A patient should *always* follow a physician's advice and additionally, ask his or her pharmacist very specific information on each individual prescription drug. Readers should not make *any* decisions about *which* drug to take based on this book. Readers and patients should talk to both their physician and pharmacist about every prescription medication they take, especially any new medication. THIS BOOK SHOULD NEVER BE USED AS A SUBSTITUTE FOR MEDICAL ADVICE. This book does *not* provide medical advice or legal advice. Rather, this book provides "consumer advice" and acts as a reference, to guide readers in asking *questions* and making more informed choices about prescription drug purchases. .

Conclusion

Prescription drugs are a very important part of all our lives. One survey showed that: <u>THREE IN FOUR AMERICANS HAVE TAKEN PRESCRIPTION DRUGS AT LEAST ONCE IN THE PAST YEAR</u>. In addition, that same survey showed that *84%* of Americans over the age of 50 have taken a prescription drug in the past year[3].

Not every American can afford life-saving quality prescription and non-prescription drugs. Cost- sharing and an increase in prices and availability are requiring some Americans to take drastic measures such as buying from Canada and Mexico. Individuals will be increasingly required to make more informed choices about their prescription drug purchases and to participate in what's known as the consumer-focused, self-care movement. Americans today need to take control over what medicines they use, how much they cost, and how they will pay for them. **Many experts have suggested that consumers should shop around and do price comparisons.**

It's even been suggested by President Bush's task force (including the Department of Health Human Services), as well as many State Attorneys General. However, this is a fairly new concept and Americans don't know where to turn. This book will be a place to begin. It will provide the knowledge required to make informed, cost-effective prescription drugs purchases. Hopefully, it will help readers in establishing thoughtful discussions with their health care providers. I look forward to the day that all Americans have access to *affordable* prescription drug therapy. In the meantime, YES, paying for the high costs of prescription drugs may be as inevitable and painful as paying taxes. However, *no one* should pay one penny more than necessary and no one should ever pay full retail price.

Good Luck and Happy Shopping!

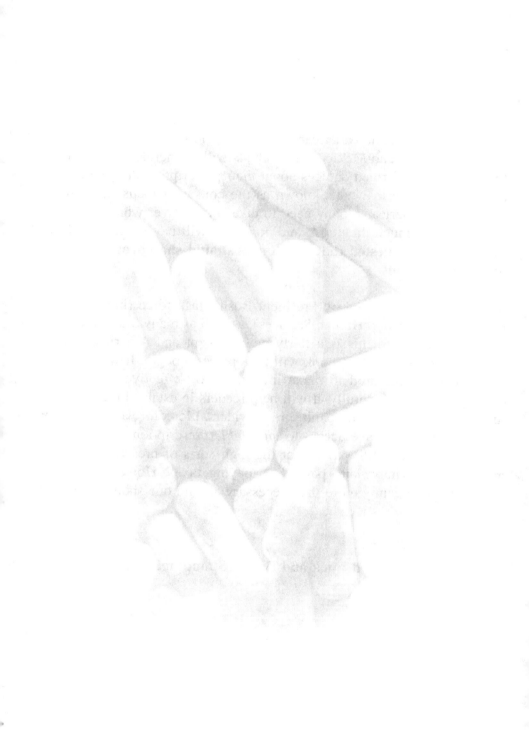

PART I   PRESCRIPTION DRUGS 101

Chapter 1
Drug Costs, Origins and Definitions

Introduction

"Would you like to save *30-60%* on all your prescription drugs?" How many times is this phrase seen in newspapers, magazines, and Internet advertisements? How reliable is the information being presented? How accurate? What about safety? How many articles does a responsible person need to read in order to obtain the facts on purchasing prescription drugs in the United States, Canada, and Mexico? Why don't most sources actually tell consumers and patients where to find the best prices?

This book will help its readers <u>save money on prescription drugs safely and responsibly.</u> The information will empower consumers and patients to make informed, yet cost-effective decisions about purchasing prescription drugs.

First, let us consider health care costs in general. Health care spending reached *$1.6 trillion* dollars in 2002, up from 1.4 trillion in 2000. Although prescription drug costs account for a small portion of the total health care dollar, (only 11%) it is one of the fastest growing components, especially in out-of pocket expenditures. Prescription drugs costs amount to 23% of out-of-pocket healthcare costs for the average consumer[1].

Prescription drug sales were estimated at **$221 billion in 2004**![2] Add to that OTC (over-the-counter) drugs, which are an additional $47 billion and dietary supplements with another $15-$20 billion. The total drug expenditures of the U.S. amount to more than 70% of the entire gross national income of the country of Switzerland! Also, compare this amount to Canada's $15.9+ billion for the same time period[3].

Why is this important to the reader? <u>One reason is the paradigm shift requiring consumers to pay more out of pocket costs.</u> This shift is being accomplished through insurance companies' tiered prescription benefit plans that incorporate different copayments for generic, brand and non-formulary products. The result is an increase in consumer cost sharing, especially in the last 5 years. (See chapter 6). The day of the $5.00 prescription copay has practically disappeared. In addition, many prescription drugs are being converted to over-the-counter (OTC) drugs that do *not* require a prescription. Many HMOs and insurers do not cover OTCs and this also contributes to higher out-of-pocket costs. Currently, prescription drug prices are based on a capitalistic pricing system, relying on supply and demand. This means that pharmaceutical companies will charge whatever they believe the market will bear.

As of 2005, some Medicare recipients (about 25%) and most of the uninsured population (approximately 40 million Americans) have been without prescription drug benefits. In other words, the most vulnerable populations have been required to pay full price for their prescription drugs. This is what sets the U.S. apart from many other industrialized countries where there is only one set price for everybody. For many, the high cost of prescription drugs is a major hardship and often requires making a choice between purchasing prescription drugs and paying the electric bill.

Why do drugs cost so much?

Many variables have contributed to the spiraling costs of prescription drugs in the past 10 years, including:
1. Americans are using *more* prescription drugs
   - In a survey conducted by the Center for Disease Control, one or more prescriptions drugs, and/or over-the-counter drugs were provided or prescribed in *544.5 million* physician office visits (66.1% of all office visits in 2000.)[4]

- The increase in the *volume* of prescriptions filled in retail pharmacies alone increased from 1.9 billion in 1992 to 3.2 billion in 2001. The average *number* of prescriptions per person per year increased from 7.3 in 1992 to 11.1 by 2001.[5]

2. The average *price* for prescription drugs is increasing.
   - In 2004, the average price for a prescription drug rose 6.5% to $63.59 from $59.52.[6]

3. There has been a shift to purchasing higher-priced brand name drugs.
   - 50 high-cost prescription drugs account for *44%* of all retail prescription drug sales, even though there were more than 9,500 drugs available. Out of the top 50 selling prescription drugs, only five were generic brands[7].

4. There are *no price controls* in the U.S. This often encourages price manipulations by the manufacturers, distributors, and pharmacies. Prescription drug costs can vary as much as 30% between pharmacies!
   Note: See *APPENDIX A* in this book for the best prices.

5. The U.S. is experiencing an *aging population* with a greater number of chronic diseases and therefore, new therapeutic agents are being created to treat those chronic diseases.
   - For example, cardiovascular-renal drugs were prescribed or provided at 15% of all office visits[8].

6. Many brand name drug companies are finding ways to extend patent protection and stall generic manufacturing. Although Congress and the FDA have adopted new legislation to close the gaps, this practice has continued to contribute to annual cost increases.

Table 1 below displays the average costs for 18 popular brand name prescription drugs. Note: 17 out of 18 cost more than $500 annually!

Rank & Name of Drug	Avg. Price per Prescription	Annualized Cost
1. Lipitor	$80.00	$960.00
2. Prevacid	$125.98	$1,511.76
3. Zocor	$85.00	$1,020.00
4. Celebrex	$88.93	$1,067.16
5. Zoloft	$80.55	$966.60
6. Paxil	$78.62	$943.44
7. Fosamax	$84.99	$1,019.88
8. Welbutrin SR	$69.50	$834
10. Zyprexa	$268.13	$3,217.56
11. Norvasc	$57.40	$688.80
12 Glucophage	$63.00	$756.00
13. Oxycontin	$189.01	$2,268.12
14 Neurontin	107.34	$1,288.08
15. Vytorin	$78.99	$936.00
16 Premarin Tabs	$27.39	$328.68
17. Nexium	$144.99	$1739.88
18. Risperdal	$153.63	$1843.56

Up to now, it has been almost impossible for the average American consumer to sort out all available information and find a way to comparison-shop for the best prices on prescription drugs. It's very hard for a patient to start thinking about shopping for discounts when he or she is doubled over in pain or is seriously ill. Consumers are usually at their most vulnerable when making prescription drug purchases.

This book will provide useful, cost-saving information. Specifically, review APPENDIX A for cost comparisons for 100+ top selling prescription drugs.

Understanding what prescription drugs can do:

Prior to beginning any comparison-shopping, it is crucial for consumers to have a rudimentary understanding of prescription drugs. Chapter 1 is "Prescriptions 101" information that provides a brief history of drug origins, nomenclature, definitions, and classifications. Subsequent chapters in Part I of this book are chocked full of vital facts about pharmaceutical companies, the FDA, HMO drug coverage, prescription discount cards, etc. With this basic understanding, the reader will gain confidence in his or her ability to comparison shop and find the best values on prescription drugs *without* compromising quality or safety.

Drug Origins

The word 'pharmacy' comes from the Greek word: pharmacon, meaning "drug." The use of drugs in healing is as old as civilization itself. Even 5,000 years ago there is evidence that garlic was used for medicinal purposes to heal, purify, and strengthen the mind, body, and spirit. Since 2800 BC, the Chinese have used ginkgo biloba to sharpen mental focus[9]. The ancient Egyptian Ebers Papyrus from 1550 B.C. lists more than 700 herbal remedies. Hippocrates, the father of Western Medicine used herbal remedies as early as the 4th century B.C.[10]

By the 18th century, pharmacology in America was making dramatic advances. The American Revolution forced American physicians and druggists to manufacture their own drugs instead of purchasing them from Europe. By 1820, the Massachusetts Medical Society printed their first official listing of drugs: "The Pharmacopoeia of the United States."[11] (All of the drugs listed were natural remedies.) Paul Erlich, a German bacteriologist, created a very well known medicine used to treat syphilis known as arsphenamine in 1907.

In fact, each culture defines itself in part by medicinal folklore. Early medications were mixed with rituals, magic, and incantations. Shamans dispensed health advice and medicinal plants/herbs.

Today, there are more than **11,000** prescriptions, over the counter and herbal remedies and *there are more than 600 prescription drugs alone sold through retail pharmacies.*

Initially, all drugs were derived from natural sources such as plants, animals and minerals. Common examples still used today include:

- insulin   (animal)
- vitamins   (mineral)
- digitalis, opium   (plant)

Most of the prescription drugs developed *today* are produced through synthetic means. Synthetics are often more effective and less toxic than naturally obtained substances. It's also easier to prepare them in standardized units. Examples of synthetics include:

- Tylenol with codeine   (synthetic)
- Prilosec   (synthetic)

An interesting example of how synthetic drugs can be created from natural sources is told in the story of the discovery of a hormone found in the saliva of a **gila monster** similar to the one produced by humans to control blood sugars and reduce appetite. A synthetic version is now on the market to assist in the management of diabetes.

However, without a doubt, the new drug revolution for the 21st century will be shaped from advances in "biotechnology" and "biopharmaceuticals." Biopharmaceuticals are a collection of technologies such as bioprocessing (which uses living cells to manufacture products such as human insulin) and recombinant DNA technology (which combines and modifies genes to create new therapies). As one can expect, biopharmaceuticals are also among the most expensive drugs available. Today, there are *120* biopharmaceuticals for sale around the world with sales of over $32 billion. Currently, biotech drugs account for 10-15% of the current pharmaceutical market and approximately 27% of the medicines in active clinical trials are biopharmaceuticals. Some exciting new biophar-maceuticals include gene therapy products and DNA vaccines.[12] Examples of biopharmaceuticals include:

- Epogen and Betaseron_
- Human insulin

In the future, biopharmaceuticals will have a revolutionary effect on our ability to treat chronic diseases on a patient-by-patient basis.

Drug Definitions

What exactly is a drug?

Under United States law, a drug is:

"Any substance (other than a food or device), intended for the user in the diagnosis, cure, relief, treatment, or prevention of disease, or intended to affect the structure or function of the body."

The Merck Manual of Medical Information, Second Home Edition, has a much more workable definition:

"Any chemical that affects the body and its processes." [13]

A drug can only provide a cure or treatment by altering or affecting the rate at which biological functions proceed; they do not change the basic nature of existing processes or create new functions. What this means is that with the assistance of pharmacotherapy, your body ultimately tries to heal itself and therein lies the mind-body-spirit connection. Prescription drugs are wonderful products but they actually work by assisting the body in healing itself.

Drug Nomenclature

Prescription drugs actually have three names:

1. Chemical: The chemical name of a drug represents the atomic or molecular structure.

2. Generic: This is the non-proprietary name for the drug. Many of the generic names are a kind of shorthand of the chemical name or structure. Sometimes a generic name will be one word, sometimes two. The second word in the name is specific to the chemical structure of the drug (also known as the salt form) that allows the drug to be made into different product types, such as liquid or tablet. When the Food and Drug Administration (FDA) approves a medication for use, it is given a generic name. Even if there is a generic name, not all prescription drugs have a generic form available to the public. There are times when a drug cannot be duplicated or there have not been adequate tests performed to prove that the generic is bioequivalent. Or simply, it is not profitable to create a generic equivalent. (Please see chapter 4 for more important information on generic drugs.)

3. Brand: The brand name is the name assigned by the U.S. Adopted Names Counsel (USAN), which is sponsored by the American Medical Association, the American Pharmacy Association, and United States Pharmacopeia. This is a proprietary name denoting a patent granted by the FDA to the drug manufacturer. The drug manufacturer can own one or more patents and can receive a patent for not only the drug, but also the delivery system (how the drug is released or distributed in the blood stream). (Please see chapter 2 for more information on the FDA approval process.)

Example of Drug Names for the common drug: Tylenol [14]

Chemical Name	Generic Name	BrandName
N-(4-hydroxyphenyl) acetamide	acetaminophen	Tylenol

Drug Classifications

Illegal drugs-

- There are many reasons for a drug to be classified as illegal. Many drugs are illegal based on their addictive qualities and/or the harm they cause physiologically.
- A drug can be legal in another country, but *illegal* here. Reasons could be political (e.g. legalization of marijuana) or procedural (approved by another federal regulatory body but not yet approved by the FDA.)
- Prescription drugs can be legal in the U.S. but still taken illegally. (e.g., no legal prescription obtained or a drug prescribed for someone else. U.S. drugs re-imported from Canada and Mexico by U.S. citizens are also considered illegal).

Legal Drugs-

Prescription Drugs-
- Also known as 'legend drugs'. Prescription or legend drugs were first established in 1951 and require a written or oral prescription by a health care practitioner licensed to prescribe this type of drug.
- The type of practitioner that can be granted privileges to write prescriptions vary from state to state, but many include physicians, nurse practitioners, physician assistants, psychologists, and dentists.

Over-the-counter (OTC) Drugs-
- OTC drugs are sold without a prescription at any local pharmacy, grocery store, Internet site, etc. The FDA determines when a drug is safe enough to convert to an OTC drug. Currently, over 700 OTC drugs available in the drugstore today were once sold as prescription drugs. In general, OTCs are much

safer and oftentimes more cost-effective than prescription drugs. However, due to easy accessibility, there are often more risks associated with taking them. (See chapter 10)

Herbal remedies and supplements-

- Herbal remedies, dietary supplements, vitamins, and minerals are all considered dietary supplements by the FDA. Recent studies show that over 15 million adults in the U.S. utilize herbal remedies and dietary supplements. It is believed that at least 30% of these adults do not disclose the use of alternative therapies to their physicians. They fear that the physicians will pass judgment or they believe it is none of their physician's business. Since by definition herbal and dietary supplements can be taken without a prescription, they have become an important component of "self-care management." This is a new trend from the last decade that has taken hold due to a more educated, informed public with access to the Internet. Many herbal remedies and dietary supplements, taken with many prescription drugs, can cause *severe* interactions and complications. However, many remedies can have remarkable curative properties and can be very effective. Remember, *all* drugs originally started as botanicals or nutraceuticals (medicines derived from natural plants and animals). Today, 25% of prescription drugs are from plants.

It is important to understand that when certain supplements such as vitamins and minerals are taken in small doses, an individual is getting the normal *physiologic* requirement. On the other hand, when taking large doses of vitamins or minerals, individuals are taking a *pharmacologic* dose.

"Schedule Drugs"

The Comprehensive Drug Abuse and Control Act of 1970 created a classification of drugs by abuse potential. The agency responsible to control drug abuse and enforce laws related to drug abuse is the Drug Enforcement Agency (DEA), an arm of the Department of Justice. In accordance with this act, "Schedules" or categories were created to classify drugs with potential abuse. The schedules or categories are listed below:

- Schedule I: Drugs with no accepted medical use, or other substances with a high potential for abuse (e.g. heroin, LSD, Marijuana, peyote).

- Schedule II: Drugs with accepted medical uses and a high potential for abuse, which, if abused, may lead to severe psychological or physical dependence (e.g. cocaine, codeine, Dexedrine, Dilaudid, Demerol, Ritalin, Methadone).

- Schedule III: Drugs with accepted medical uses and a potential for abuse less than those listed in Schedules II, and I, which if abused, may lead to moderate psychological or physical dependence (e.g. Tylenol with Codeine, certain barbiturates).

- Schedule IV: Drugs with accepted medical uses and low potential for abuse relative to those in Schedule III, which, if abused, may lead to limited physical dependence or psychological dependence relative to drugs in Schedule III (e.g. Librium, Valium, Ativan, Phenobarbital, and Darvon).

- Schedule V: Drugs with accepted medical uses and low potential for abuse relative to those in Schedule IV and which, if abused, may lead to limited physical dependence or psychological dependence relative to drugs in Schedule IV (e.g. Robitussin A-C syrup.)

Anyone taking prescription drugs listed in the examples above should be aware of the very real potential for abuse. Patients should *always* discuss the risks vs. benefits with their health care professionals prior to beginning drug therapy. If a reader believes he or she is taking a prescription drug that may be Schedule 1-IV, but does not see it listed above, the reader should check with his or her physician and/or pharmacist and ask about side effects, abuse potential and alternatives.

How Are Drugs Priced?

Often American consumers don't understand how pharmaceutical companies can charge $4 a pill when it's universally known that the cost of production was probably a penny. The pharmaceutical industry always responds the same way: *high prices are a byproduct of Research and Development (R & D.)*

So how does it work? Every prescription drug product that makes it to market has to cover the R & D expenses for the 5,000 that did not. It is estimated that the R & D costs for each new prescription drug are in the neighborhood of $200-$800 million. However, an independent third party has never substantiated these figures. In addition, roughly half of the $800 million consist of "opportunity costs," which is money that would have been made by the drug developer if the R & D funds had been invested in equities.

As seen from the pie chart below, the majority of the cost of prescription drugs goes to the manufacturer.[15] (For a more detailed discussion, see Chapter 5.)

Total Price: $63.59 in 2004

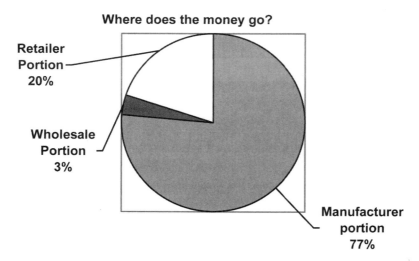

Where does the money go?

Retailer Portion 20%

Wholesale Portion 3%

Manufacturer portion 77%

Total Price: $63.59 in 2004

Two of the three drug pricing components comprise four primary sources; the raw-material supplier, the drug manufacturer, the sales and marketing business and the company that sells the drugs to a pharmacy (known as a wholesaler, distributor or dealer). A price is then established called the Average Wholesale Price or AWP, as a means of price comparison and communication. The AWP is similar to the Average Retail Price used in the garment industry. After an AWP is assigned, pharmacies then add a dispensing fee. Usually, the pharmacy assigns a set fee for all prescriptions- for example $5.00- regardless of the prescription costs. Pharmacy fees are "hidden" in that they are not billed separately and are included in the total price.

With all the controversy regarding drug prices, some states are now requiring that the cost of the medication be added to the labeling (e.g., it is required in New York). Other states voluntarily post prices for the top 20-50 most commonly prescribed prescription drugs. In addition, prescription drug prices for seniors on Medicare are now available at www.medicare.gov. This information, when available, will assist consumers in making more cost-effective choices. In addition, cost information for the top 100+ prescription drugs are included in Appendix A of this book, with updates available at www.prescriptionpathway.com.

Chapter 2
The Food and Drug Administration (FDA) & Clinical Trials

TIP: Wondering if your expensive drug is going generic (less expensive) soon? Want safety tips from the FDA? Log on to www.fda.gov for more information

So why do prescription drug products cost so much and does the FDA have an effect on drug pricing and availability? Moreover, why should Americans care about the FDA?

To help answer these questions, this chapter is devoted to understanding the FDA (Food and Drug Administration) and what role it plays in the who, what, when, where and why of prescription drug costs.

Introduction

The primary source for monitoring the manufacturing and distribution of prescription drugs is the Food and Drug Administration (FDA). The FDA is a behemoth of a government agency under the umbrella of the U.S. Department of Health & Human Services. Federal Regulations for food and drugs in the U.S. dates back to the 1906 enactment of the Federal Food and Drug Act.

The FDA is the "Enforcer and Safety Officer" for Americans. However, the FDA and the government do not enforce price controls and they will be the first to tell U.S. citizens that they are not responsible for prescription drug pricing. Nevertheless, there is a legitimate argument that, by virtue of all the federal rules and regulations, the FDA does *contribute* to the high costs of prescription drugs. In fact, many consumer groups, as well as a few government officials, would like to see the implementation of price controls for prescription drugs in the U.S.

Let us consider:

1. The FDA oversees $1.5 *trillion* dollars worth of products every year (including both food *and* drugs). Twenty cents, or 20% of every dollar Americans spend each year are for products regulated by the FDA. By its very size, the FDA is a very powerful force to reckon with.

2. The FDA grants or denies approval of all applications for new drugs and biologicals and thus acts as the "gatekeeper" for all drug products in the following classifications:
   • Prescription Brand name drugs
   • Prescription Generic drugs
   • Over-the-counter drugs

3. The FDA can also withdraw pharmaceuticals from the marketplace if post-marketing surveillance suggests that the public health risks outweigh the benefits. For example, ephedra products were banned in December 2003 due to concerns over cardiovascular effects, including increased blood pressure and irregular heart rhythm. Prescription drugs, OTC products, and herbal supplements containing ephedra and ma huang were banned in 2004.

4. It costs somewhere between $200-$800 million to develop a new prescription drug, largely due to the FDA approval process (more about this later in this chapter).

To begin to understand how the FDA implements its gatekeeper functions, and how this effects pricing, it is important to first understand the FDA approval process. This includes how drugs get to market, how long it takes, and the "fail safe" procedures in place to protect the public.

The FDA approval process- Clinical Trials

In 2003, the average time to create, approve, and get a new drug to market was *13 years and 3 months*, five months longer than in 2002. Three drug products actually took up to 25 years.[1] One reason for the long approval process is the extensive 3-4 phases of clinical trials required for each new prescription drug.

The drug approval process actually begins *before* FDA involvement. It begins as a "hunting expedition" when scientists screen hundreds of thousands of molecules against specific diseases for which they wish to focus their time and attention and resources. First, approximately 10,000 compounds are investigated and from that, over 5,000 compounds are tested! (As of March 2004, there were 6,525 active products being studied.)[2] Of that number, only <u>5</u> will probably make it to the human-test stage. For every <u>5</u> medicines that enter clinical trials, only <u>one</u> survives the three phases of research.

According to Jonathan Wilkin, M.D., a medical officer at the FDA: "There is a lot of serendipity in drug development."[3] Indications for use are often completely accidental and unexpected. For example, one drug intended to treat depression also seems to take away the desire to smoke. As a result, this drug, a slow-release form of buproprion, marketed as Zyban, was approved as an aid to smoking cessation treatment.

In addition, we now have "biotech products." Biotechnology drugs are described as drugs that are produced from living organisms. The worldwide biotech market is now worth over 37 billion and accounts for 27% of the total active drug pipeline. And the biotech market is big business. Currently, the seven biotech products among the top 50 drugs reported combined sales of 15.1 billion worldwide![4]

According to the drug companies, there are currently 1,000 pharmaceutical and biotech drugs in the pipeline.

Pre-clinical Research: Animal Testing

Once the sponsor finds a compound(s) with promise, drug development begins with testing for the drug's toxic pharmacologic effects through "in vitro" and "in vivo" lab animal testing. 'In vitro" is a term meaning the drug's effects are monitored in an artificial environment *outside* the living organism: e.g. "an egg fertilized in vitro." While 'in vivo" is a term indicating that the entity was studied *inside* a living organism.

At this stage, the pharmacological profile of the drug is studied to determine the acute toxicity in a least 2 species of animals. These early tests are usually resource-intensive and require significant investment in product synthesis, animal use, laboratory analyses, and time. The short-term toxicity studies range from 2 weeks to 3 months depending on the proposed duration of the use of the substance in the proposed clinical studies. The process can take 1 year or more.

The whole purpose of this phase is to demonstrate that the drug can be safely tested in humans. Once this is determined, the sponsor can then move on to the 4 phases of the clinical trials process. According to the FDA, fewer than 10 percent of INDs for new molecular entities progress beyond the investigational stage.

FDA and Clinical Trials-Phase I-IV

After the pre-clinical research is completed, a sponsor files an Investigational New Drug Application (IND) with the FDA. The IND allows the sponsor to begin the 3-4 phases of the clinical trials process that is required by the FDA prior to selling a prescription drug in the U.S.

The four phases of FDA approval are:

Phase 1:   This is the phase that includes the *initial* trials on *healthy* humans, conducted in volunteers. Phase 1 studies test the safety, tolerance, and pharmacokinetics of the compounds (i.e. absorption, distribution, metabolism, and excretion of the drug). Phase I also investigates the side effects that occur as dosage levels are increased. For each individual, this initial phase of testing typically takes several months. The total number of subjects included in Phase 1 is generally just between 20-80 people. The complete Phase 1 process usually takes a couple of years. About 70% of experimental drugs pass this initial phase of testing.[5]

Phase II: Phase II studies are well-controlled and closely monitored trials that test the compound in patients with the *condition the drug is intended to treat.* Dose and dosing regimens are explored, often to establish upper and lower boundaries. Short-term side effects and risks associated with the drug are also monitored. Phase II studies usually involve several hundred people and can take a year or more.

Phase III: These are usually the final human trials required by the FDA. Just like Phase II, the trials provide safety and efficacy data in patients with the condition the drug is intended to treat, but do so in *large* enough numbers so that the results can be extrapolated to the general U.S. population. The two trials may include several hundred to several thousand people and can take 3 years or more. Enough data is collected in the phase III trials to complete the labeling and prescribing requirements. Phase III trials can be either controlled or well controlled. The FDA generally requires *two* randomized, well-controlled, double-blinded trials with proof of safety and efficacy. A randomized, controlled trial indicates that there is a randomly selected group taking the investigative drug as well as a randomized control group that is taking other drugs or a placebo (sugar pill). "Double-blinded" indicates that neither the physician nor the patient knows which participants are receiving the drug and which are receiving the placebo.

Phase IV: Phase IV studies occur <u>after</u> a drug is approved. They may explore such areas as new uses or new populations, long-term effects, and/or how participants respond to different dosages. It used to be that Phase IV trials were rare; trials were designed to compare the *investigative* drug with existing drugs (s) in the same therapeutic class, when a pharmaceutical company believed that their drug was superior to those already on the market. However, now that more drugs are "fast tracked" from priority reviews, the FDA requires more post-marketing Phase IV trials. Phase IV trials may also be required if certain safety issues surface about the product after it is approved. The FDA has requested post-marketing commitment studies in 73% of the approvals for new drugs from 1998-2003. However, according to recent data from the FDA, only 33% of post-marketing drug studies are proceeding on schedule![6]

Phase 0: This is a new proposed category for use in exploratory IND applications, which would enable drugmakers to conduct various exploratory studies *without* being limited by Phase 1 trial rules. Drug sponsors would be able to choose between multiple molecular entities rather than be limited to a specific one.

How much does FDA approval cost?

The FDA approval process is the primary contributor to the cost of discovering the new drugs which has been estimated to cost anywhere between $**200 million to $800 million** (depending on which study can be believed). If the average cost of R & D is in fact in the middle at around $403 million, which is more likely, then 1/3 to ½ of that amount is probably connected to clinical trial related expenses. However, other estimates of typical clinical trial costs for a series of Phase I, II, and III involving 3,300 patients would bring the cost of clinical trials from between $6.6 million to $22.1 million[7]. In addition, there are other fees payable to the FDA for the marketing applications (NDAs), etc. which are above and beyond the cost of the clinical trials.

The "NDA"

When a sponsor of a new drug believes that there is enough evidence of the drug's safety and effectiveness to meet FDA's requirements for marketing and selling the news drug, the sponsor submits a New Drug application (NDA) for new drugs or a Biological License Application (BLA) for new biologics. The application must contain enough data from specific technical viewpoints for a thorough review, including chemistry, pharmacology, medical, biopharmaceuticals, and statistics for a decision to be made. If the FDA approves the NDA, then and only then can the drug be marketed in the U.S.   The sponsor usually applies for an NDA or BLA after successful completion of their Phase III studies.

A continuing problem has been that relatively few new NDAs are approved on the "first cycle" They are submitted with incomplete information and thus require 2, 3, or even more cycles. The FDA is now focusing on decreasing or even eliminating the multiple cycles by planning more formal communication procedures with the sponsor along the review process. This would drastically decrease the amount of time it takes to receive FDA approval for a new drug.

Accelerated and priority drug reviews

The FDA may grant an "accelerated drug review" or "priority review" for drugs that will treat a disease or condition where there are indicators-called surrogate endpoints-that can allow the FDA review teams to reasonably predict that the drug will provide some benefit. With an accelerated drug review, the manufacturer is required to continue testing *after* FDA approval, to demonstrate that the drug indeed provides therapeutic benefits for the patient.

Under an accelerated review process, drugs can be made available to the patients before general marketing begins, usually *during* Phase III trials. An excellent example of the success of this program was the approval of protease inhibitors used to treat HIV infections. All of the protease inhibitors were approved in a matter of months and one was approved in only 42 days. The decline in AIDs-related deaths in the US is partly attributed to the availability of these drugs.

As of 2004, the FDA has also expanded the Accelerated Drug Review process to include drug products for obesity and diabetes. Although these conditions may not be immediately life threatening, they are at epidemic proportions in the U.S.

Better than a sugar pill

The American public may not realize that: in order to get FDA approval, a drug only has to show that the improvement made by the drug is statistically significant when measured against a *placebo*, (sugar pill). It does not have to be as good as or better than other drugs already on the market. An example is a recent study for a new estrogen therapy patch introduced in 2004. According to unpublished data, after 2 years of treatment, bone density increased an average of 3% with the new patch, compared to an average of .4% in the placebo group. However, other drugs already on the market such as Fosamax and other non-hormonal drugs (bisphophonates) already increase bone density 5% or 6%.

However, good news: As of September 2004, the U.S. Senate set aside $15 million for government research to compare the effectiveness of prescription drug products *against each other*. The funding will pay for the Department of HHS's Agency for Healthcare Research and Quality to research "outcomes, comparative clinical effectiveness and appropriateness of prescription drugs and other healthcare items."

Pharmaceutical companies *pay* the FDA for their approvals

The FDA collects user fees from the pharmaceutical companies that submit the NDAs. The theory behind this is that since the industry is receiving a service from the government through the review of the pharmaceutical company's marketing applications, then the industry should contribute directly toward the costs of the review process. In exchange for these fees, companies are given assurances that the FDA will examine applications more quickly. Due to this process, the review times have indeed been cut in half. However, many believe this practice automatically instills a conflict of interest and provides a monetary incentive to approve drugs that may be less than efficacious. Consider that the Bush

Administration is requesting funding of $1.49 billion for the FDA for the Fiscal year 2005. But *added to that* is the amount expected from drug companies in user fees -an additional $350 million. This is obviously a substantial portion of the entire budget (19%), which in turn helps pay the salaries of many of the reviewers, and thus establishes an automatic conflict of interest.

FDA Timelines

The FDA approval process is an important discussion for this book because it is usually blamed for the high cost of prescription drugs. For example, of the $80/month a patient pays for Lipitor at the local drug-store, 77% of the retail price goes to the drug company. According to the pharmaceutical industry, a large portion of that 77% is for R & D, of which the FDA approval process is the most expensive component.

With this very comprehensive approval process, it's easy to see why it can take *an average of 13+ years* between early laboratory testing and FDA approval. Some of the drugs, especially biotech drugs, may take from 15-25 years to make it to market. For example, Epogen, the first biotech chemotherapy drug, took over 25 years before it was available for purchase in the U.S., due to R & D, politics and other business con-siderations.

Many informed consumers argue that they have *already* paid for this R & D process with taxpayer dollars and this argument has merit. A report by the Joint Economic Committee of Congress in 2000 showed that: "The federal government, mainly through the National Institutes of Health (NIH) funds about 36% of all medical research. Of the 21 most important drugs introduced between 1965 and 1992, *15* were developed using knowledge and technologies from federally funded research using tax payer dollars."[8] This amounts to more than *$23 billion* taxpayer dol-lars each year.

Patents & Exclusivity

Patents

Patents and exclusivity work in a similar fashion but are distinctly different. However, both processes ensure profits for the sponsors of new drugs while intentionally delaying the availability of less expensive generic drugs.

Patents are granted by the U.S. patent and trademark office. Although this is not a responsibility of the FDA, the patent process affects the FDA's ability to approve generic drugs. If a drug is patented, other companies cannot manufacture the drug, make a generic substitute, or be subject to market competition. Patents can be granted anywhere along the development lifeline of a drug. Patents usually expire <u>20</u> years from the date of filing. This means the patents can expire before drug approval or years after the drug is on the market. Additional patents can be filed at any time after, given that drug development can be an ongoing process.

There are 4 types of pharmaceutical patents:

1. Composition of matter,
2. Method of use,
3. Formulation and
4. Manufacturing

In general, the two strongest types of patents for a compound are composition of matter and primary care of use.

It's been no secret that pharmaceutical companies have been accused of using patents as a way to delay generic versions which in turn directly contributes to the high cost of brand name drugs. There are many strategies deployed, including what is called "evergreening" patents on an aging product. Evergreening means listing multiple patents and filing patent infringement lawsuits against generic firms in order to extend the exclusivity as long as possible and delay generic competition for years.

Sometimes the patent is challenged based on just on one chemical compound (metabolite) produced in the liver as it metabolizes the prescription drug for use in the body. How does this work? The primary chemical change that drugs undergo in the body takes place in the liver and it works like a chemical factory to not only make substances needed by the body but also to break down other chemicals. So once in the liver, the drug may break down completely and then move through the blood for circulation in the body or it may break down into a smaller, different chemical called a metabolite. Some metabolites have pharmaceutical benefits just like the active drug, while others just continue through the bloodstream until they are further reduced and then reused or eliminated. The pharmaceutical companies' have used the metabolite argument to seek new patents and/or extensions.

There are many examples of the abusive use of patents, but a few mentioned here are directly quoted from an excellent book written by Fran Hawthorne called *The Merck Druggernaut*.

Examples include:[9]

- "The blockbuster allergy medicine, Claritin, was set to expire in December 2003. Schering-Plough sued potential generic makers, claiming that they would violate a separate patent on the chemical compound (or metabolite) called DCL that is produced in the liver when the pill is swallowed."

- "Bristol-Myers Squibb tried a similar "metabolite defense for its anti-anxiety drug BusSpar three times in 1999 and 2000 which was due to go off patent in November 2000."

- "For its diabetes medicine Glucophage, Bristol-Myers tried to obtain a 3-year patent extension by combining two of the exclusivity regulations (6-month pediatric extension, 3-year extension for new usages), and another legal provision concerning the labeling...."

- "AstraZeneca attempted to delay generics for Prilosec, insisting that generics would violate the patent on the *process* it used for making the drug."

Sometimes, rather than challenge a patent and drag the resolution through the courts, the pharmaceutical companies will come out with a newer "improved" version of the same drug. Then they will market that drug as having either a better side effect profile or better clinical outcomes such as when Clarinex was used to replace Claritin and Nexium was used to replace Prilosec.

Readers who want to know if the prescription drugs they are taking are ready to go off patent can check for a drug product's patent expiration dates on www.fda.gov/cder, then click on "Drugs@FDA," then write in the name of the drug and hit 'enter'.

Types of exclusivity:

Exclusivity, on the other hand, is granted upon approval of a drug product when statutory requirements are met. Exclusivity was designed to promote a balance between new drug innovation and generic competition. Since it can take 12-15 years to get a drug to market, the financial investment must be made *prior* to marketing. The exclusivity means that the sponsor then has approximately 5-12 years to make up the R& D costs and to make a large profit before a competitive generic version can be approved.

Protection	Description	Duration
5-yr Hatch-Waxman	Granted to new chemical entities (NCE). If no unexpired patents are listed with FDA, generics can file after this exclusivity expires.	5 years from date of approval
3-yr Hatch-Waxman	Granted to modified version of existing drugs with new clinical data (e.g. new dosage form, new clinical use). This applies only to the modification of the product. Generics can file at any time, but cannot be approved until exclusivity expires	3 years from date of approval
Orphan Drug	Granted to drugs with indications with less than 200,000 U.S. patients. (There are over 6,000 rare diseases that afflict 25 million Americans). Protects against both generic and other branded versions.	7 years from date of approval
Pediatric extension	Granted in exchange for pediatric studies for a drug as requested by FDA	6 months added at date of approval
First-to-file exclusivity for generics	Generic exclusivity granted to the earliest generic application prior to expiration of listed patents from the brand version. No other generic versions can be approved during this exclusivity	180 days from date of commercial launch or court decision declaring patents invalid or not infringed

Table 1. Exclusivity Source: CMS and FDA.

The U.S. grants five years of exclusivity for new branded prescription drugs (plus an additional three years for modifications of the brand name drug and 6-month for the pediatric extension). This means that generic firms are prohibited from filing for a generic drug application until the 4th year of the exclusivity period. Patents and exclusivity may or may not run concurrently and may or may not encompass the same claims, but exclusivity is _not_ added to the patent life. Interestingly enough, the European Union is now voting to pass legislation that would give European companies _11_ years of exclusivity before facing generic competition.

Delaying generic competition is a lucrative business, especially when dealing with a blockbuster drug (a blockbuster drug is one that has over $1 billion in sales per year). Consider that _70%_ of all drug sales in 2001 were from just 50 drugs. Pharmaceutical companies can pocket hundreds of millions more dollars by delaying generic competition, even _after_ paying court costs to fight the generic competitors. (See Chapter 5).

Moreover, while *exclusivity* legislation was probably needed initially to foster innovation, the pharmaceutical industry has become very adept at "gaming the system." They receive the 5 year exclusivity, then add a new dosage form-usually a once daily dosing- and then receive another 3 years exclusivity and then do a pediatric study, receive *another* 6 months and finally, fight the generic companies in court to extend exclusivity while the case is being heard. The exclusivity process can force the high cost of the drug to continue for 8-10 years! On top of the 5-year exclusivity, for instance, there is the wait for the generic firm to receive their final approval after they have filed, which typically takes an additional 12-18 months. All of these delays contribute to the high cost of drugs, especially the innovative new brand name prescription drugs.

How many new drugs are approved each year?

Now that we have discussed all the regulations and the costs involved in getting new drugs approved, is it making a difference? The big question is: *has the number of new drugs increased over the years and has the federal regulations helped in approving costs as well as accessibility?*

Actually, no. Although approval *times* have indeed improved, the *number* of *new* drugs approved (known as new molecular entities or NMEs) by the FDA has remained constant or even declined. The total *number* of *all* approved drugs has not increased either. During the 90s, about 30 drugs with new active ingredients were approved each year. In the 2000s, that number dropped to the 20s.

Fortunately, the number of biologics has continued to increase by 25%. In 2003, the FDA approved 21 (NMEs) and 25 new biologicals. Among the 21 new *pharmaceuticals* in 2003, two were new drugs to compete with Viagra for the treatment of erectile dysfunction and one was yet another cholesterol-lowering statin. These types of new drugs are sometimes known as "me too" drugs, which means they are very similar to the drugs already on the market. Some readers might find it surprising that *seven* of the 21 were developed by European companies and that the number of new NMEs from Europe was expected to increase to 14 in

2004. Only 2 of the 21 NMEs in 2003 are expected to be blockbuster drugs. It remains to be seen whether these numbers will increase in 2004 and 2005. The FDA is attempting to increase the number of approved drugs by streamlining the approval process so that prescription drugs, especially generics, can be approved on the first cycle. More generics were approved in 2004 (474) and at a faster rate (15.7 months), but this was partly due to the upsurge in generic submissions.

What does it take to remove a drug from the US market?

Some say that in its effort to fully review data associated with adverse events, the FDA is too slow in acting when a drug has been linked to serious illnesses and deaths. For example, the drug Serzone, which was taken off the market in Europe in 2003, was still available in the U.S. in 2004. Although it was not actively marketed or shipped by the original drug manufacturer, it was still available, both in the original brand as well as in a generic version.

Off-label use

There are many prescription drugs that have off-label uses. An off-label use is one in which the drug is prescribed by a physician to treat a *different* disease or symptom other than the one(s) approved by the FDA. Many times a drug is found to treat a disease very different from the one originally studied and sometimes it happens by accident. Examples of off-label uses include many cancer treatments.

FDA laws that affect drug approval and pricing

Even though the FDA does not control drug prices and the U.S. has long resisted implementing price controls, there are at least three FDA regulations that really affect drug pricing. They are:

    1.   Food and Drug Cosmetic Act (FDCA)-(1938): This act was passed to require all drugs to be proven *safe* before being market-

ed, thereby initiating a system of drug regulation in the United States. At the time, the basic definition of "safe" under this act was "nontoxic." This act was originally passed as the result of 107 deaths of Americans who had taken a sulfa drug laced with poisonous solvent.[10] The FDCA basically started the effective monitoring and licensing of prescription drugs. In addition, the FDCA is the law most cited by the FDA when making its claim that importing drugs from another country is illegal.

2.   Prescription Drug User Fee Act (PDUFA) – (1992): PDUFA was enacted by Congress to shorten the approval process. The PDUFA encourages an accelerated approval timeline, not only for new drug applications, but also for all stages of the drug development process.   PDUFA encourages communications between the FDA and the pharmaceutical companies, particularly before Phase III.   In 2002, the PDUFA required the FDA to act on 90% of the new drug applications within 10 months. The act has served to speed up the process so that an average approval time for priority applications dropped from 21 months to 6 months. Standard drug reviews have fallen from 27 months to 19 months. According to the Health and Human Services Office of the Inspector General, FDA employees who responded to a survey about the review process felt that it had deteriorated over the past 5 years due to shorter review times. However, the respondents did not feel that the time constraints resulted in any threat to the public health and this has not been empirically proven.   Due to the PDUFA, "user fees" are used to monitor drugs after they reach the market.

3.   Prescription Drug Marketing Act (PDMA)-(1987): The PDMA was enacted in response to concern over safety and competition issues raised by secondary markets for drugs. The PDMA prohibits the reimportation of a drug into the US by anyone except the manufacturer. This is the other statute most commonly cited for justification of the prohibition of individual reimportation.

4. <u>Drug Price Competition and Patent Term Restoration Act</u> (known as the Hatch-Waxman Act)-(1984)- This may be the one most important pieces of legislation to affect the modern pharmaceutical industry because it locks in all the exclusivity described in Table 1 of this chapter. It was enacted to balance the competing interests of the brand name and generic industries and to streamline the process for getting generic drugs to market.

5. <u>Medicare Modernization and Improvement Act</u> (MMA)-(2003). The MMA was the sweeping legislation passed in 2003 to provide prescription drug coverage for seniors and the disabled, but it actually involves much more than just paying for drugs. It also closes some Hatch-Waxman loopholes, including a new patent rule, which limits brand firms to <u>one</u> 30-month "stay" when a generic drugmaker challenges a patent in court.

The Prozac story

A good illustration on how legislation and regulations can affect the profits of a drug is revealed with the Prozac story. The FDA approved Prozac in 1987. At the time, it was the quintessential breakthrough treatment for depression, creating a popular class of antidepressants called SSRIs (selective serotonin reuptake inhibitors). Through patent and exclusivity provisions, the drug company was able to extend its chokehold on generic competition until August 2001 - <u>14</u> years *after* the drug was approved. Delaying generic competition allowed the drug company to make <u>billions</u> of extra dollars and forced consumers to keep paying the high price of over $3 a pill! As soon as generic versions were available, the Company saw its quarterly earnings decrease by 20%.[11]

Clinical Trials

Consumer participation in FDA clinical trials has become an important component of the approval process. The more consumers participate, the faster the timelines for approving life-saving, innovative pharmacotherapy. Both healthy individuals, as well as patients with specific diseases, can participate in clinical trials.

In 2003, 200,000 research professionals managed clinical trials that included over *1 million* Americans. According to CenterWatch, a Boston-based patient information group that monitors the clinical trial industry, there are currently over 6,000 new therapies being tested in 80,000 locations around the country.[12] Globally, an estimated 60,000 clinical trials are being conducted.

Although some individuals may have concerns that participating in a clinical trial might not be safe, the actual statistics of anyone being harmed is very small. According to the FDA, only 1 in 10,000 patients have died from the effects of drugs being studied.

Not only is participation in a clinical trial an altruistic undertaking, but it can also be profitable. <u>Fees for participation in a Phase I study can range from $25 to $1,500 per person.</u>

In the past, most prospective treatments and drug products would be tested at a major university or at an elite research center such as the National Institutes of Health or the Mayo Clinic. Typically, a pharmaceutical company would find what is considered a "marquee scientist" to lead the charge. The human subjects for the trial would come from the center's pool of patients or referrals. However, with increasing treatments in the pipeline, more volunteers were found to be needed. For the last decade or so, over half of the clinical trials have involved physicians in private practices and other health care facilities; here the same regulatory standards for good practices and human subject protection apply. The sponsor or company must obtain approval from an Institutional Review Board, which is usually composed of both physicians and lay people and the Board is charged with determining that the patient's rights are protected.

It is also becoming increasingly common for the drug companies to work with contract research organizations (CROs), which oversee the operations and hire "monitors" at each site to make sure protocols are strictly followed.[13]

Informed Consent

Anyone entering a clinical trial in the U.S. must sign what is called an Informed Consent. Informed Consent is a form indicating that the patient understands what will happen to him or her during the study. If the patient is a child, a parent or guardian must sign the form. The informed consent will provide details on the nature of the study as well as the risks involved. This form will contain information such as what treatment will be given and what kind of problems might occur. It will also tell the patient what costs are covered by the study and what costs might need to be paid for by the patient or the patient's insurance company.

Questions a patient should ask before participating in a clinical trial

Before deciding to participate in any clinical trial, patients should ask the following questions:

1. How long will the trial last?
2. Where is the trial being conducted
3. What treatments will be used and how?
4. What is the main purpose of the trial?
5. How will the patient safety be monitored?
6. Are there any risks involved?
7. What are the possible benefits?
8. What are the alternative treatments besides the one being tested in the trial?
9. Who is sponsoring the trial?
10. Do I have to pay for any part of the trial?
11. What happens if I am harmed by the trial?
12. Can I opt to remain on this treatment, even after termination of the trial?[14]

In addition, patients should *always* discuss clinical trial participation with their health care professionals prior to enrollment.

Be aware that in order to participate as a healthy volunteer in a Phase I trial, patients must not be taking any medications that could cause confounding factors in the study results. For example, a healthy male in his 20s might still be excluded in a clinical trial if he has taken medications for depression, ADD or a mild chronic condition.

If patients already *have* a disease and would like to determine if there are any experimental drugs being studied that could help their condition, there are two reliable sources: the patients' personal physicians and/or a credible website that includes a registry.

Three very good websites include:

1) www.clinicaltrials.gov: This federal website created in 1997 contains a government-maintained database with over *11,000* government and industry trials. This source provides patients, families, and members of the public easy access to information about the location of clinical trials, their design and purpose, criteria for participation, and, in many cases, further information about the disease and treatment under study. *Clinicaltrials.gov is probably the most comprehensive website for anyone interested in participating in a clinical trial.*

2) www.clinicaltrials.com: This is a privately maintained website and is often accessed by mistake due to the similarity of its name with the government's web address at clinicaltrials.gov. It contains a listing of current clinical trials and other general information.

3) www.centerwatch.com: This commercial website also contains a broad listing of commercial and academic trials. It provides links to several clinical trials matching services, which help match the interested party to a specific trial. In addition, general information in the trials process is provided, such as the twelve questions listed above.

Registering and reporting clinical trials-cracks in the foundation

The FDA *requires* sponsors of new clinical trials to submit information to the FDA within 21 days from the start of enrollment. This information or guidance covers all studies conducted under FDA IND regulations for new drugs to treat serious or life-threatening diseases, including foreign trials and both publicly and commercially funded research. Recently, pharmaceutical companies were chastised for non-compliance because only <u>49%</u> of the trials had been registered! And while there is only a very small concern with actual harm coming to a clinical trial participant, there is a much larger concern about whether the clinical trial *results* are accurate and shared with the appropriate authorities. High profile investigations abound concerning 1) the lack of reporting negative results, 2) FDA approval of drugs on shaky clinical trial results and 3) the lack of truthful reporting by the clinical researchers themselves. A story was published in 2003 about a cardiologist who falsified research data and was found by the FDA to have "repeatedly or deliberately submitted false information and repeatedly or deliberately violated regulations" in comparing aspirin with another drug in heart patients. Rather than ban this cardiologist from ever participating again in clinical trials, he received an insignificant punishment and was only restricted to leading just two FDA-regulated clinical trials for three years!

Other grave examples of alleged acts of omission or fraud in clinical trial reporting include studies on SSRI medications for depression in children and the inattention or alleged concealment of the trial results for VIOXX.

To combat all of these problems, Republican Senator Henry Waxman proposed the FACT Act (Fair Access to Clinical Trials), which would **require** results of clinical trials, good or bad, be posted on the National Institutes of Health federal website. The bill did not pass. The American Medical Association has also called for the HHS to establish a comprehensive registry of clinical trials. At the present time, the <u>www.clinicaltrials.gov</u> website is acting as this registry. While it was originally developed by the National Institutes of Health to alert the public about *current* clinical trials in which they could participate, it now also includes Phase III trials that are no longer recruiting. Currently, it also includes post-marketing trials and will complement the FDA's new MedWatch postmarket surveillance system.

PhRMA, the pharmaceutical's trade organization has also developed a website to post clinical trial results: www.clinicalstudyresults.org. However, there are less than 20 records in the entire database, and since it is voluntary, it will probably never be comprehensive. Several individual drug companies are also developing their own websites to post clinical trial results.

In addition, the International Federation of Pharmaceutical Manufacturers and Associates (IFPMA) is launching an internet search portal in the fall of 2005 that will provide a centralized location to access clinical trial registries and databases worldwide.

Moving clinical trials to third-world countries

Some of the large pharmaceutical manufacturers are now moving human clinical trials to low-cost countries in order to decrease R & D costs. According to the FDA, one large pharmaceutical company has estimated it could save more than $200 million annually in R & D costs if the trials were conducted in countries such as India and Poland. This company currently has more than 70,000 patients enrolled in clinical trials. A 30% shift to other countries could save $10,000-$15,000 for each patient enrolled and could free up $200 million or more annually for the company's R & D budget.

It is estimated that in two years *many* of the Big Pharma will conduct 50% or more of their clinical trials outside the U.S. What remains to be seen is if the savings will result in new drugs for consumers, a decrease in the cost of new drugs, or just higher profits for the pharmaceutical industry.

Conclusion

The FDA assures the safety of our drug products by monitoring the development, manufacturing, and distribution methods, yet there is still much to be done. For example, one of the FDA's monitoring activities includes 3,500+ FDA inspections a year at manufacturing facilities to ensure that strict standards are met. However, documentation shows that currently there are *delays* with over half of the reviews. The budget for FDA inspections is also expected to decrease, not increase, in 2005.

FDA can and should improve its entire system. Many argue that the FDA approval process is too costly, too prolonged, and lacks objectivity. Many have called the FDA too "accommodating" or too "cozy" with the pharmaceutical industry and there appears to be many conflicts of interest built into the system. Congress, medical groups, advocacy groups and the FDA itself are trying to improve the internal processes.

Republican Dan Burton of Indiana has been quoted as saying that "the FDA needs to do some innovative, 'out of the pillbox' thinking." While Rep. Burton was speaking about the ban on drug imports, the statement can actually apply to many of the FDA responsibilities going forward.

In the meantime, Americans need to understand that every time a patient purchases an expensive brand name drug such as Lipitor or Celebrex at the local drugstore, they are paying for many cost components. They are not only paying the costs to conduct research and development, but also the FDA approval costs, the costs for all the drugs that *didn't* make it through the approval process, and lastly, the costs of drugs *yet to be discovered.* While the reasons may be clear, it does not make the bitter pill any easier to swallow for Americans who are without prescription drug coverage.

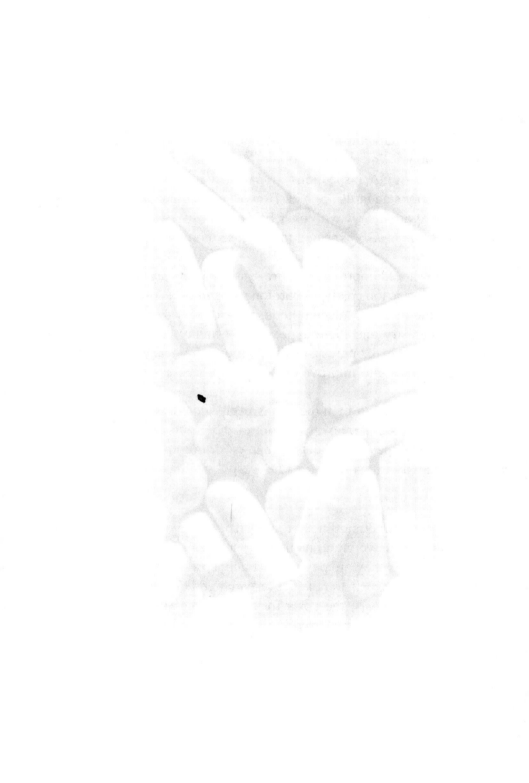

Chapter 3

Drug Safety and Counterfeit Prescription Drugs

> TIP: To find the latest information on counterfeit drugs, check the website www.prescriptionpathway.com, Use your user ID and password at the end of this book to gain access to the website.

Introduction

Remember old man Gower, the pharmacist in the Christmas movie, "It's a Wonderful Life"? As the story goes, a drunken Mr. Gower who is overcome with grief due to a telegram announcing the death of his son in WWII, mistakenly mixes a patient's pills with poison. Jimmy Stewart's character-George Bailey-, is a young boy working in the pharmacy who recognizes the mistake and warns Mr. Gower (and is slapped in the face for it!) Young George Bailey, by this simple action, prevented a potential lethal situation.[1]

While risks similar to the one depicted in this classic Christmas movie have been greatly reduced in the 21st Century, taking a prescription drug is never without some risk. The general belief is that *if* the drug product is on the market, it must have been proven that the healthcare *benefits* of taking the drug outweigh the *risks.* Moreover, most of the risks involved in taking a prescription drug are not due to the drug itself. In fact: THE #1 PROBLEM IN TREATING ILLNESS TODAY IS THE PATIENT'S FAILURE TO TAKE PRESCRIPTION MEDICATIONS CURRECTLY.

However, "caveat emptor" or buyer beware! In today's world, there are a broad variety of risks associated with taking prescription drugs. Individuals, armed with knowledge and a healthy dose of skepticism, must be ever vigilant and responsible for their own safety.

Risks associated with taking prescription drugs include:
- Side effects
- Drug interactions and/or contraindications
- Distribution problems that lead to counterfeiting, adulteration, improper storage
- Packaging and labeling
- Dispensing the wrong medicine and/or the wrong dose

Who is Responsible for Drug Safety?

Our country's safety procedures are among the best in the world. Despite recent news attention to prescription drug safety following the recall of the drug VIOXX, as well as the media coverage about antidepressants increasing the risk of suicide in children, approximately 77% of Americans still feel confident about the safety of prescription drugs sold in the U.S.[2]

However, with the increase of counterfeiting, criminal activities, and fraudulent national and international Internet companies, the types of risks, as well as the volume, have been altered and in many cases worsened.

This chapter will address what the medical community is doing to improve the drug supply as well as what <u>YOU, the reader,</u> can do to protect yourself.

There are 3 major groups responsible for ensuring the safety of the prescriptions drugs purchased in the U.S.:
1. The Food and Drug Administration (FDA)
2. Your individual health care providers (includes pharmacists)
3. **<u>YOU</u>**- Be Vigilant!

Number 1: FDA (Food and Drug Administration)

The FDA and its federal safety regulations exist today to protect the public. Chapter 2 discussed the protections for the development of drug.

What has not yet been discussed are the less than perfect rules and regulations for reporting possible side effects, illnesses, and even deaths caused by prescription drugs. Surprisingly, pharmaceutical companies are <u>not</u> obligated to warn patients about side effects, and complications; they are only required to warn physicians (who are considered the learned intermediary) and the FDA.[3]

Drugmakers are also <u>not</u> required to report cases of counterfeit products to the FDA. However, through the drug industry's trade organization, Pharmaceuticals Manufacturers of America (PhRMA), many drug companies voluntarily report suspected counterfeit cases to the FDA within 5 days of discovery.

What this means is that while the FDA is ultimately responsible for safety, by the time the public has learned about the problems, many patients have already been exposed. This is why it is important to have healthcare providers; pharmacies *and* consumers do their part.

Number 2: Healthcare Providers and Pharmacies

A. Problems

Physicians, hospitals, and pharmacies have implemented many safety systems to ensure the safe distribution and administration of prescription drugs. However, in the general course of healthcare services administration, mistakes *do* happen. Here is a sample of some of the safety problems facing the healthcare industry:

1. Medication Errors:
   Consumers are already aware of the large number of medication errors as statistics are reported in newspapers and magazines. There are many reasons for medication errors but primary causes include:

   - Brand and generic names for drugs that look alike or sound alike
   - Similar packaging and design.

The U.S. has made progress over the past few years in finding methods to decrease medication errors, but probably one of the most effective ways has been the implementation of voluntary patient safety reporting programs that allows for individuals and institutions to admit problems and collect objective, comprehensive data. The United States Pharmacopeia (USP), a non-profit, non-governmental organization, operates two principal programs: the Medication Errors Reporting (MER) program and MEDMARX^{SM}. These are two of the four private sector programs available for reporting drug/medication errors. MEDMARX^{SM} is an Internet-accessible and anonymous medication error reporting program used by more than 775 hospitals and health systems to anonymously report and track medication errors. MER, presented by USP in cooperation with the Institute for Safe Medication Practices, is a nationwide program used by health professionals to report medication errors confidentially and anonymously. With a national database, healthcare professionals can monitor medication errors, looks for patterns and trends and work together to find solutions.

2. Handwriting

As many patients know, physicians are notorious for bad handwriting. Pharmacists are quite adept at reading and deciphering their words on prescription forms, but still medication errors occur, especially when so many drug names are similar. Illegible handwriting has caused medication errors both in hospitals as well as retail pharmacies and the consequences can be lethal. Some states have passed laws requiring physicians to write the condition or disease on the prescription form in order to provide a checks and balances system.

B. Solutions and Information

1. Electronic Prescribing- This is the practice of using computers, usually PDAs (small handheld personal data assistants) to prescribe medications, as opposed to paper prescription forms. By

communicating with pharmacies electronically, the prescription information is more reliable, legible, secure, and less prone to abuse than paper prescriptions. Electronic prescribing reduces handwriting errors, lost orders, and enters prescriptions in data bases so that dangerous drug-drug interactions can be identified before a drug is prescribed. In addition, the physician can check whether the drug he wants to prescribe is covered by a patient's insurance *before* the patient leaves the office. Studies have suggested that electronic subscribing could save as much as $27 billion per year, yet only 5-18% of physicians and other clinicians are using electronic prescribing systems.

2. FDA's "MedWatch"

MedWatch is a program created by the FDA to serve as the Safety Information and Adverse Event Reporting Program. Basically, it is a public health safety outreach program for both healthcare professionals and their patients. MedWatch collects reports from health professionals *and consumers* regarding prescription and non-prescription drug adverse events, quality problems, and counterfeiting and medication errors. This enables the FDA to share timely, accurate unbiased and useful safety information on prescription drugs and other medical products. One problem that exists with this system is that, due to the fact that it is *voluntary* reporting, it is estimated to pick up no more than 10% of serious side effects.

To report adverse effects, drug problems or medication errors:

- Log on to www.fda.gov/medwatch and select "Submit Report" or
- Call 1-800-FDA-1088 (1-800-332-1088) to submit report by phone
- Reporting is strictly confidential

While MedWatch should be the optimal reporting solution, there have been several cases in the past few years where drug companies have failed to report appropriately. There are steps underway to make sure that MedWatch is fully utilized, including a pro-

43

posed rule that would require all Rx drugs and certain OTC products to include MedWatch's toll free telephone number on each drug product. By including the phone number on the drug label and/or patient information sheets, *consumers* would have the information readily available and could be responsible for reporting adverse drug events as they happen. The MedWatch information would state: *Call your doctor for medical advice about side effects. You may report side effects to the FSA at 1-800-FDA-1088.* Pharmacies could comply with this rule by attaching a sticker to the container, using a preprinted prescription vial cap, or by distributing a separate sheet of paper or the appropriate FDA-approved medication guide on which the instruction has already been printed. This information would be provided for both new prescriptions as well as refills.

3. FDA's "Drug Watch"

A new program known as "Drug Watch," appearing on the FDA web page, was created to identify drugs for which the FDA is actively evaluating early safety signals. The Drug Watch is *not* intended to be a list of drugs that are particularly risky or dangerous. Rather, inclusion of a prescription or OTC drug on the Drug Watch signifies that the FDA is attempting to assess the meaning and potential consequences of emerging safety information. The Drug Watch page can be viewed at www.fda.gov. No one is quite sure what effects this program will have; however, drug companies are especially worried that it will lead to increased litigation and/or unsubstantiated claims.

4. FDA's Drug Safety Oversight Board (DSB). This is component of the FDA's new drug safety initiative in 2005. It is in its infancy stage and very little information is available at the present time. For more information, readers should see the author's website at www.prescriptionpathways.com.

5. Drug Counseling

Pharmacies are required by the Centers for Medicare and Medicaid Services (CMS) to offer prescription medicine counseling to Medicaid patients and to review their medicine usage. (Note: mail-order pharmacies must provide toll-free telephone service in order to meet this requirement.) Since pharmacists are *required* to a do the drug counseling for Medicaid patients, most pharmacies have expanded the policy to include *all* patients; in fact, many states have passed laws to give all patients the legal right to counseling. This has led to better education for consumers. If a pharmacist asks a patient if he or she has ever taken a medicine before and if he/she has any questions, the patient should not be so quick to say no. Counseling by pharmacists can include important aspects of the medicine such as its description, dosage forms, length of treatment, special directions, side effects and most importantly, drug-drug interactions, food-drug interactions, etc. A couple of minutes of counseling allow patients to ask *crucial* questions, such as the "DARK" questions listed below. Whether patients are afforded the opportunity to ask the questions at the doctor's office or not, pharmacists can *still* provide vital additional information and answer many questions related to both prescription and non-prescription drug products.

6. <u>Labels:</u>

The FDA-approved label is the official description of a drug product. This applies to drug labels for both prescription *and* over-the-counter medications. Labels include:

- What the drug is used for
- Who should take it
- Adverse events (side effects)
- Instructions for uses in pregnancy, children, and other populations and
- Safety information for the patients

Labels on the pill bottle should contain the following information:

a. Date when the prescription was filled,

b. Serial number of the prescription,

    c. Name and address of the pharmacy, name of the patient,

    d. Name of the prescribing physician,

    e. Directions for use,

    f. Auxiliary labels such as whether to take with food,

    g. Name of medication,

    h. Name of drug manufacturer,

    i. Quantity of the drug,

    j. Expiration date,

    k. Initials of the licensed pharmacies and

    l. Number of refills.

NOTE: These are *FDA* requirements, so labels from drugs purchased in Canada or Mexico may be different.

7. Patient Information Sheets:

The information provided on a printed sheet, monograph or leaflet at the pharmacy contains labeling information, but is written in nonprofessionals' terms so that consumers will read and understand it. The "Action Plan" prompted these printed sheets for the Provision of Useful Medicine Information. The requirements for the printed sheets are that they include the medicine's uses approved by the FDA, directions for use and possible side effects. They must be scientifically accurate, unbiased, specific, complete, understandable, up-to-date, and useful. According to federal regulations, this information was required to reach at least 75% of patients by the year 2000 and at least 95% of patients by 2006. *Almost all* of the major chain drug stores, supermarket pharmacies, mass merchandisers, and the independent pharmacies are now compliant with offering this material. Along with receiving counseling at the pharmacy, this material should be a consumer's first and primary step to understanding the medicine he/she is taking. However, consumers should understand that the information on the patient information sheet is an *abbreviated* version of the labeling/package inserts information.

8. Package Inserts:

A Package inserts or "PPI" is the full prescribing information included by manufacturers with the prescription products. Legally, the PPIs are extensions of the labeling information. Readers who have received drug samples from doctors' offices have received PPIs- they are usually multi-folded sheets about the size of a couple of postage stamps and are written in very tiny print. Patients may also see them accompanying a prescription for contraceptives and estrogens. The popular Physicians Desk Reference, or PDR, that is used by many consumers and health-care providers alike is actually a compilation of PPIs.

9. Drug Guides

Drug Guides or medication guides are the 600-1,200 page books available on bookstore and drugstore shelves. They contain drug safety information for the most common drugs prescribed. Drug guides are great tools and include a wealth of information, but can often be intimidating due to their size and medical language Remember, most of the information contained in the drug guides is required by the FDA and must also be provided at the time a patient fills a prescription. However, the drug guides are still use-ful because the information sheets, inserts, and labels on bottles can be confusing or be misplaced. In addition, a single PPI or information sheet will *not* address possible interactions with all the prescription, non-prescription, and herbal supplements that are specific to each patient. This is where the drug guides may be particularly useful. They often include supplemental information such as a generic cross-reference, a price "score," etc. If a con-sumer is interested in purchasing a drug guide, here are a couple of excellent ones:

1. Adderly, Brenda D, M.H.A. "The complete Guide to Pills," The Ballantine Publishing Group, 1997, NY, NY.
2. "PDR," 52nd Edition, Oradell, NU: Medical Economics 1998. See www.medec.com

10. **Free** from the FDA

Prescribing information can also be obtained *free,* if you have access to the Internet. The FDA's Center for Drug Evaluation and Research (CDER), (who is responsible for evaluating drugs before they are sold), offers consumer medical information sheets based on the package insert on *all* prescription and OTC drugs approved since *1998.* For more information, visit the website: www.fda.gov/cder. Then click on "Drugs@FDA" and type in the name of the drug. Next, click on the name of the drug and an overview page will appear. Click on the drug name to view "drug details" and then click on "label information."

11. Brochures from the manufacturer/drug company

Beware of the drug information in the form of a leaflet or brochure from the drug's pharmaceutical company, as their marketing material can be misleading. There have been many cases of warning letters from the FDA to drug manufacturers about this very problem. The information from the pharmacy or the FDA web site listed above (Drugs@fda.gov) and/or a reputable drug reference guide is more accurate.

Number 3: You

Studies show that up to *half* of the people who use medicines do not use them as prescribed.[4] Considering that more than 3 billion prescriptions were filled last year, this number is staggering. Fortunately, most results of misuse do not result in serious injuries. However, misuse can actually be very costly in the long run; both to consumers and to the health care system.

There is a cacophony of information available to the public on how to safely take medications. In fact, perhaps there is *too much* information available from too many credible and non-credible sources because this can cause confusion or inaction. This chapter attempts to highlight some of the best consumer safety information available, which may very well save a life, as well as save money.

Knowledge is the best weapon in ensuring the safety of consumers and their families. The best place to begin when it comes to safety precautions is with a knowledge and understanding of the actual prescription form written for a prescription drug(s).

A correct prescription form (slip) will look something like this:

Doctor's Clinic 9999 E. Main Street Broadway, Arizona	DEA #:
Pt. Name_____ Address_____	Age: _____ Date: _____
Rx: Serax 30mg #15 Sig. i tid prn	Refills: ___ times
_____ Dispense As Written	_____ Substitution Permissible

Patients should *keep a copy of each prescription form for two reasons*:

    1) It is easier to call pharmacies to comparison-shop with a copy of the actual prescription in hand *prior* to filling the script. (If a patient cannot read the handwriting, he/she should ask the physician or other health care professional in the doctor's office to print the name of the drug on their insurance form.)

    2) With a copy of the original prescription, a patient can compare the information on the label of the pill bottle with the information on the prescription form to ensure they are prescribed the *correct* drug. If the

names do not match (e.g. patient is given a generic but is not familiar with the name), the patient should ask for an explanation from the pharmacist.

Safety Information

The Agency for Healthcare Research and Quality (AHRQ) and the National Council on Patient Information and Education (NCPIE) has developed a comprehensive, yet easy to understand guide concerning safety information.[5] *I recommend that readers review this information <u>before</u> reading any future chapters in this book!* It outlines "<u>Four Ways to Play it Safe</u>" which are listed below, along with a few editorial comments:

1. Give Your Health Care Team Important Information: Tell them about:
   - Prescription medicines you already take.
   - Medicines you buy without a prescription (OTCs) such as aspirin, laxatives, and cough medicine.
   - Vitamins and dietary supplements such as St. John's Wort or gingko biloba.

2. Also, tell your health care team about:
   - Allergies to any medicines or if you have had problems when taking a medicine before.
   - About any other doctors or health care professionals who have prescribed. medicine for you or suggested that you take a vitamin or herbal supplement.
   - If you are pregnant, may get pregnant or are nursing a baby.
   - About any other illness you have, like diabetes or high blood pressure.
   - If cost is a concern, there may be another medicine that costs less that will work the same.

3. Get the Facts about Your Medicine

- Be informed- ask questions about every new prescription medicine. Get the answers you need from your health care team *before* you take your medicine.
- Read the Prescription- If your doctor writes your prescription by hand; make sure you can read it. If you cannot read your doctor's handwriting, your pharmacist might not be able to either. If your doctor submits your prescription to the pharmacy electronically, ask for a **copy of the prescription.**
- Know what your medicine is for- Ask your doctor to write down on the prescription what the medicine is used for.... Not just, "take once a day," but "take once a day for high blood pressure." - And keep a **copy of your prescription**!
- Ask Questions- by asking questions now; you may be preventing problems later. If you have questions before your doctor visit, write them down and bring them to your appointment. For a list of questions; see *** following page:

4. Stay with Your Treatment Plan

- Take your medicine as prescribed. If for some reason you do not want to take all your medicine, (e.g. you have side effects), call your health care provider and ask for advice, *before* you stop taking it. He/she may be able to prescribe a different amount or a different type of medicine.
- Ask your doctor if your prescription needs to be refilled. If you are taking a medicine for high blood pressure or to lower your cholesterol for example, you may be using it for a long time. If the prescription does need to be refilled, ask the health care provider for two scripts: one for the first 30 days and then another for the refills. (This way, you will be able look for more cost effective choices later, such as mail order or Internet pharmacies.)
- Ask whether you need blood tests, x-rays, or other lab tests to find out if the medicine is working, to find out if it is causing any problems and to see if you need a different medicine. Ask your doctor to tell you what the tests showed.

- Never give your prescription medicine to somebody else or take prescription medicine that was not prescribed for you, even if you have the same medical condition. Although this is a very common practice, it can be a very dangerous one! There are so many reasons a medicine might not be right for you – drug interactions with some other medicine you are taking, allergic reactions, other health conditions, etc.

5. Keep a Record of Your Medicine

- Always keep a record of the "medicines" you are taking. "Medicines" includes prescription drugs, over-the-counter drugs, vitamins and other dietary and herbal supplements. (See section below)

*** Referenced on the previous page:

Questions to ask your Doctor about your medicines:

1. What are the brand name and generic name of this medicine?
2. Can I take a generic version of this medicine?
3. What am I taking this medicine for?
4. Does this new prescription mean I should stop taking any other medicines I'm taking now?
5. How do I take the medicine and how often do I take it? If I need to take it 3 times a day, does that mean to take it at breakfast, lunch, and dinner, or to take it every 8 hours?
6. Do I need to take it all, or should I stop when I feel better?
7. How long will I be taking it? Can I get a refill? How often can I get a refill?
8. Are there any tests I need to take while I'm on this medicine?
9. When should I expect the medicine to start working? How can I tell if it's working?
10. When should I tell the doctor about a problem or side effect?
11. Are there foods, drinks (including alcoholic beverages), other medicines, or activities to avoid while I'm taking this medicine?
13. What are the side effects that can happen with this medicine?
14. What should I do if I have a side effect?

15. What happens if I miss a dose?
16. What printed information can you give me about this medicine?

Want a quicker, shorter list to safety (and low cost)?
Remember: D A R K

The information listed above is a lot to remember. If it helps, this author has created an abbreviated version. It is known as "**DARK**":

At the **D**octor's office **A**sk:

D_____o I have any conditions or medications that would keep me from safely taking this drug? (Then discuss all your health problems and hand the physician or pharmacist your "Checkbook Medication Record." Make sure you have included all vitamins, minerals and herbs you take, as well as all over-the-counter and prescription drug products.)

A_____m I being prescribed a generic, and if not, why not?

At Home, **R**ead and **K**now:

R_____ead the safety information that accompanies the prescription. Look for possible drug interactions, contraindications, etc.

K_____now what condition/disease the drug intended to treat. **Keep** a copy of the actual prescription. (This allows you to check the name of the prescription on the prescription slip with the name on a pill bottle to ensure that you received the right prescription.) Remember that each drug may have two names- a brand name and a generic name. Note: if you don't have a copier at home most grocery stores, drugstores, and discount stores have a copier available at the customer service desk so you can make a copy of the prescription *before* taking it to the pharmacy window.

Medication Record

BE SURE TO LIST ALL DRUG PRODUCTS ON A MEDICATION SHEET OR RECORD. THE FORM IN THIS BOOK IN APPENDIX C IS RECOMMENDED. This form can be torn out and slipped in a person's checkbook so that it is available at all times. Although it is not as comprehensive as some other forms, the "KISS" (Keep It Simple Stupid) principle can be applied here. If patients use a form that is a separate piece of letter-sized paper that requires patients to remember to pack it each time they go to a doctor's office and pharmacy, odds are they will not have it with them when they need it. *However, be advised that patients with a long list of medications with varying dosing schedules may need a more sophisticated form.* Even then, though, the checkbook form can still be used to alert the patient's health care providers and pharmacists for the need to obtain more extensive medication records. So many of the safety problems associated with taking prescription drugs are due to taking the medications incorrectly or taking certain medications together (i.e. drug-drug interactions). The Checkbook Medication Record in this book will help the patients, doctors, and pharmacists in checking for complications and interactions.

Safety of dietary and herbal supplements

Dietary and herbal supplements are a big business in the U.S., with sales estimated at $20 billion and over 16,000 products available! Dietary supplements (which includes herbal and botanical supplements, vitamins, minerals and amino acids), are marketed under the provisions of the Dietary Supplement Health and Education Act (DSHEA) of 1994. Regulated as foods, *most* dietary supplements are available under a grandfather provision of that act. Unlike prescription and OTC drug products, marketing firms, and/or manufacturers are not required to produce any pre or post marketing safety or efficacy data for dietary supplements. Rather, the burden of proof falls on the *FDA* to prove that the products are not safe once they have been available to the public for a very long time. Only then can dietary supplements that were "grandfathered in" be removed from the market (e.g. ephedra products.)

Only manufacturers creating and marketing new dietary ingredients in the U.S. *after* 1994, that are not recognized as a food substance or otherwise are present in the food supply, must demonstrate to the FDA that the ingredient is safe for use in a dietary supplement.

While most vitamins and minerals are considered very safe in normal doses, herbal supplements can be very dangerous, especially if they trigger interactions with specific prescription and non-prescription drugs. According to Lane Johnson, M.D., Associate Professor at the University of Arizona, "unlike medications, there is no guarantee that what is *listed* on the bottle is what is *in* the bottle, or is at a dosage that is even remotely therapeutic."[6] *Please be aware that there are literally hundreds of prescription and OTC drugs that can potentially interact with herbal medicines* (for example, Siberian ginseng can increase the effects of insulin, digoxin; and hormone therapy.) It is recommended that readers who are taking or considering taking any herbal supplements talk to their healthcare professionals about possible drug interactions or other complications. Another great source to find out more about drug interactions between herbal remedies and prescription drugs is the book is: "A Pocket Guide to Herbal Remedies" by Lane P. Johnson, M.D., MPH.

Non-Profit Organizations-Public Citizen

Non-profit organizations, with no known conflict of interests, are excellent sources of drug safety information. They are a valuable component of the health care checks and balances system. One such organization that devotes all its time and attention to prescription drug safety is Public Citizen, a non-profit organization based in Washington, D.C. Public Citizen has over 150,000 members and represents consumer interests through lobbying, litigation, research, and public education. Since its founding in 1971 by Ralph Nader, the organization has become an excellent source of prescription drug safety information.

Public Citizen has published a book to provide up-to-date safety information on new prescription drugs. They are also active in legislative matters such as recently suing the FDA over the agency's failure to act on a petition it made to remove Serzone from the US market. Serzone is a drug that continues to be sold here in the US, (despite 54 cases of liver failure and 20 deaths in 10 years) but has already been taken off the market in Europe and Canada.

In addition, Public Citizen also releases a list of drugs, which can cause life-threatening reactions, or of great potential harm to patients if used together.

According to the experts at Public Citizen, the nineteen pairs of drugs, which *may* cause life-threatening reactions if used together include:[7]

Propulsid with Biaxin
Insulin with Inderal
Warfarin (Coumadin) with Tagamet
Sporanox with Propulsid
Prozac with Desyrel
Lanoxin with Calan SR
Tagamet with Dilantin
Zocor with Posicor
Hismanal with Paxil
Mevacor with Lopid
Tegretol with erythromycin
Calan SR with quinidine
Theophylline with Tagamet
Demerol with Nardil
Aldactone with potassium
Seldane with erythromycin
Butazolidin with Orinase
Nardil with Laradopa
Inderal with Tagamet

Readers should check with their healthcare professionals if they are taking any of the combinations listed above. *Important: however, readers should never discontinue a medication without speaking to their physicians first!*

For more information on Public Citizen, readers can visit their website at www.worstpills.org.

Counterfeit Prescription Drugs

Introduction

ACCORDING TO U.S. OFFICIALS, ONE IN 10 DRUGS SOLD
WORLDWIDE IS A FAKE, GENERATING ABOUT $32 BILLION IS
SALES. In fact, in some countries, 20-90% of all drugs are counterfeit!
Counterfeit drugs found in the _U.S._ has greatly increased the past few
years, with the number of FDA counterfeit drug cases growing from only
6 in 1997 to 58 cases in 2004. By 2004, there were 76 open investigations. In 2003, a total of 32 people were arrested and 25 convicted of
conspiracy to introduce counterfeit drugs into commerce.[8] Although the
number of counterfeit cases in the U.S. remains less than 1% of the total
prescription drugs sold, it is still very worrisome.

Counterfeiting drugs can be the perfect crime since the "evidence is
destroyed," literally, when the patient consumes the drug. This happens
when drugs are diluted, mislabeled, or adulterated. Counterfeiting, as
described by the U.S. government in CFR, Title 21, Sec 201 g2, means:
"a drug which on the container or labeling of which, without authorization, bears the trademark, trade name, or other identifying mark, imprint,
or device, or any likeness thereof, of a drug manufacturer, processor,
packer, or distributor other than the person or persons who in fact manufactured, processed, packed or distributed such drug and which thereby
falsely purports or is represented to be the product of, or to have been
packed or distributed by, such other drug manufacturer, processor, packer or distributor." Adulteration, described by the FDA is "to make impure
by adding extraneous, improper, or inferior ingredients." This can alter
the breakdown or delivery of the drug as well as making it superimpotent
(i.e. _too much_ of the active ingredient) or more commonly, subpotent (i.e.
not enough of the active ingredient). Counterfeit drugs may also be
deliberately and fraudulently mislabeled.

The 1987 Prescription Drug Marketing Act was approved to safeguard drugs through the distribution process, which is where most drug counterfeiting/ tampering takes place. The law requires states to license wholesalers and prohibits hospitals or pharmacies from reselling the drugs to anyone but the patients. In addition, the law requires wholesalers to have a "pedigree paper." A pedigree is a legal document that tracks shipments from manufacturer to dispensing pharmacy. However, due to successful lobbying on the part of wholesalers, this aspect of the law has never been enforced.

Chain of Custody

The primary "chain of custody" or the route that prescription drugs take from the manufacturer to the patient is as follows:
1. Prescription drugs are made and packaged by the manufacturer –then-
2. They go from the manufacturer to an authorized wholesaler, which then distributes the medicine to retail pharmacies-then-
3. The pharmacies then sell the prescription drug products directly to the consumer.

However, several steps may be added if 'secondary wholesalers' repackage them or sell them to another wholesaler. (In some states, there are more wholesalers than pharmacies!)

Problems

In the U.S., counterfeiting problems usually occur when the drug products travel from the authorized wholesale to a "secondary or smaller wholesaler." There are more than 8,000 wholesale companies comprising a $140-billion industry. Although an estimated 46% of prescription drugs are shipped straight from the manufacturers to hospitals and large pharmacy chains, 54% are shipped to wholesalers. Of the 54%, 90% go to the three largest wholesalers in the country, which together, distribute more than $100 billion worth of drugs. The rest of the drugs are sold through *secondary* markets and that is where most of the counterfeiting problems come into play. In order to combat the problems with smaller wholesalers, the National Association of Boards of Pharmacy (NABP) is offering the Verified-Accredited Wholesalers Distributors (VAWD) program to accredit wholesale drug distributors. This can be a valuable program if pharmacies step up and choose to order only from accredited distributors. Currently, it is still just a voluntary program. (However, some states such as Florida and Nevada are starting to pass stricter laws regarding wholesalers.)

Some of the drugs that have been known recently (the last 2-3 years) to have counterfeit versions or batches are:

a. Serostim- Serostim, a human growth hormone, is used in treating some of the symptoms of AIDS and costs approximately $7,000 a month. Counterfeit serostim was discovered at two pharmacies in California in 2001.

b. Lipitor-Counterfeit Lipitor was repackaged by a company called Med-Pro and sold to at least two wholesalers in Lexington, Nebraska in May/June 2003 (nearly 200,000 tablets!) Part of the reason the pills were identified as counterfeit was due to their unusual bitter taste.

c. Procrit- Procrit, a drug used to treat cancer and dialysis patients, is a target for counterfeiting due to its high costs. Counterfeit Procrit was found to have ingredients *20* times lower than the amounts described on the labels and contained vials filled with tap water. In addition, the expiration dates were changed. The counterfeit samples of Procrit were sold nationwide and the counterfeiter walked away with 46 million!

d. Zyprexa- Zyprexa tablets, used to treat schizophrenia, were tampered with by replacing the active ingredient with aspirin. Aspirin therapy can be deadly if a patient is already taking another blood thinner. Counterfeit Zyprexa was found in 2001 in four states-Michigan Illinois, Minnesota, and Wisconsin.

e. Lipitor- Counterfeit from an Illinois repackager- Alliance Wholesale Distributor- was found to include incomplete, missing, inconsistent, and duplicate repackaging records, old expiration dates, etc. The FDA identified more than 4,500 bottles of counterfeit Lipitor.

f. Human growth hormone-HGH, sold by a dietary supplement wholesaler, possessed a Schedule I (addictive) drug. The wholesaler sold the drugs from 1999-2001 from two companies he controlled as well as from the website www.genapharm.com. What is even more surprising is that he had previously been convicted in 1998 for counterfeiting drug labels and yet was back on the streets in the counterfeiting business less than a year later!

g. Ten drugs moving through the state of Florida from 2001-2003 were counterfeit. In 2003, Florida had nearly *1,400* primary and secondary wholesalers. Counterfeit drugs found in Florida included: Procrit, Epogen, Serostim, Zyprexa, Diflucan, and AIDs drugs: (Combivir and Retrovir). This totaled *$20 million* worth of adulterated pharmaceuticals.

h. Four websites that allegedly sold counterfeit versions of Ortho Evra transdermal patches in 2004 were: www.usarxstore.com, www.europeanrxpharmacy.com and www.generic.com

i. Viagra- Counterfeit Viagra was discovered in two pharmacies in California in July 2004. A consumer discovered the counterfeiting by noticing differences in the packaging as well as unusual specks in the pills. Fortunately, the counterfeit pills did not contain any harmful ingredients. (See pictures in this chapter).

Note: None of the cases listed above involved true Canadian imported drugs; instead, the drugs were tampered with right here in the U.S! This does not mean however, that drugs being shipped from other countries are free from counterfeiting. In fact, many feel that importation would just give counterfeiters the ability to contaminate the drug supply even earlier in the process. While this had not been proven from any known Canadian imported drugs as of January 2005, it is impossible to know for sure, because the drugs are used and then eliminated, all without being analyzed.

HOWEVER: During a government's seizure in 2004, drugs imported from *Mexico* by Americans were found to be counterfeit (in this case, subpotent). The drugs were Merck's Zocor and a generic painkiller called carisoprolol. Americans purchased the counterfeit drugs at Mexican border town pharmacies. After conducting tests on the products, the FDA determined that the counterfeit Zocor did not contain *any* active ingredient! The counterfeit painkiller differed in potency (i.e., subpotent). There have been many other cases from Mexico that led to serious injury and even death; some of them are discussed further in Chapter 15.

Consumers can report suspected **counterfeiting** (and errors) by doing the following:

- Log on to www.fda.gov/medwatch and select "Submit Report" or
- Call 1-800-FDA-1088 to submit report by phone
- Note: Reporting is strictly confidential

Solutions to counterfeiting

1. Consumers/patients: The best solution to the counterfeiting problem is caution on the part of individuals. Consumers should always purchase prescription drugs from reliable, respected sources. Consumers need to be on the lookout for any irregularities in the labels, size, color, or shape of the packages of prescription drugs or in the pills themselves. In addition, consumers/patients should watch for unanticipated side effects. Everyone should be mindful of the fact that most of the drugs that are counterfeited are the *brand name* drugs that are the most costly because those are the ones with the greatest profits (e.g. Viagra, Lipitor, and Procrit.) Counterfeiters do not usually bother with generics- there isn't enough money in it.

2. Counterfeit Drug Task Force. The FDA created a counterfeit task force in 2003/2004. It includes manufacturers, wholesalers, retailers, pharmacists, consumer groups, and others. They report that there is no "magic bullet" available to stop the flow of counterfeit drugs. Both the task force, as well as private researchers

such as those at the Massachusetts Institute of Technology (MIT), have proposed such things as radio-frequency tags (see below), identification tags, electronic readers and an Object Name Service, modeled along the lines of the Domain Name Service, a software interface and an electronic product code information server.

3. Paper Pedigree: The Prescription Drug Marketing Act of 1987 that was discussed in Chapter 2 includes a requirement to implement a paper pedigree that would give a full accounting of where the drug has traveled from manufacturer to pharmacy (see chain of custody above: sometimes the drug can change hands five or 6 times). However, it appears the adoption of this rule will be delayed again until 2007, while the manufacturers attempt to adopt *electronic* pedigrees rather than paper pedigrees. It is estimated by some that it will take at least *five years* to resolve all the technical, legal, regulatory, and financial issues needed to implement the electronic system. In the meantime, the FDA and the state/ federal governments have made strides in the following areas as outlined in #4 through #9 below.

4. Bar Codes: As of February 25, 2004, the FDA finalized a rule requiring bar codes on labels of prescription drugs and biological products. Many consumers have noticed them on the label of their little pill bottles or on the boxes of OTC products sold at grocery stores and drugstores. The bar codes are similar to those on food packages and are now required on most prescription drugs and OTC drugs. Bar codes include such items as the NDA number, lot number and expiration date. The rule also requires machine-readable information on container labels of blood components intended for transfusion. The FDA estimates that the rule will help prevent nearly 500,000 adverse events and transfusion errors and save over $93 billion in health costs over 20 years! (Now, if only the U.S. could just find a way to funnel this $93 billion back into R & D for prescription drugs).

5. Blister packs: Blister packs are drugs that are individually sealed in doses by the manufacturer for amounts typical for most prescriptions. For example, a blister pack would have a 30-day sup-

ply of cholesterol-lowering pills or a 10-day supply of an antibiotic. Blister packs would eliminate one of the most problematic safety areas: repackaging. Only about 20% of the nation's drugs are now shipped in individually sealed packs and most of this is done for hospital use or for drug samples made for distribution to healthcare professionals;[9] However, this practice is quite common in some European countries. Making the blister packs childproof, but still usable for the elderly is a challenge, but again, the pharmaceutical companies have been doing it for years with drug samples. Blister packs will also require a costly distribution system.

6. Radio Frequency Identification (RFID): The FDA believes the routine tagging of products by radio frequency identification (RFID) is feasible by 2007. RFID could be an effective way to track and trace drugs from point of dispensing. RFID places electromagnetic chips (no bigger than a dot) and tags containing a unique serial number onto cartons and individual drug products. The Vanderbilt Children's Hospital in Nashville Tennessee completed a study in 2004 using RFID for expensive capital equipment. The hospital tagged its pediatric critical care equipment with RFID chips and tracked it with RFID readers, security cameras, motion detectors, and alarm detectors. This same premise can be used for tracking prescription drugs and several hospitals have begun pilot testing the RFID system. The pilot tests have categorically identified various implementation issues. It is estimated that RFID will cost 30-40 cents a package once, and if, it is implemented.

7. The shortest and safest "Custody Chain:" The more that the extra steps of the custody chain can be eliminated, (e.g. where drugs are sold to secondary manufacturers and repackaged), the less likely that the drugs can be tampered with by counterfeiters. Since consumers have little knowledge on *where* the prescription drugs come from when they purchase them, it is up to the government and the manufacturers to respond appropriately. One such measure is voluntary or state mandated certification of wholesale companies.

8. <u>Other counterfeiting technologies:</u> Other important anti-counterfeiting technologies include color-shifting inks, holograms, and chemical markers incorporated into a drug or its label. While some of these strategies might seem extreme, many experts believe these high tech solutions will pay off in the long run, both financially as well as in saving lives.

9. <u>Clinical trial results websites:</u> Just recently, both the *large pharmacy manufacturers,* as well as many *state governments,* have begun to post results of clinical trials and/or evidenced-based reports based on clinical trial reviews. Both types of websites include safety and/or efficacy information. Although both types of sites are worthwhile, the Big Pharma websites always pose the risk of biased information by either omission or by excluding information about other drugs that compete in the same therapeutic class. Consumers planning to take a prescription drug(s) for any length of time should review these websites in order to obtain safety information, warnings, and contraindications. The websites include:

   a. Eli Lilly currently posts clinical trial information on eight of its best-selling drugs on its website: <u>www.lillytrials.com,</u> with other drugs available on the site by 2005.

   b. GlaxoSmithKline was the first pharmaceutical company to post test results of their drugs at <u>http://ctr.gsk.co.uk/welcome.asp.</u>

   c. More pharmaceutical companies are expected to follow suit.

   d. Governments are posting information derived from the Drug Effectiveness Review Project (DERP), a 12-state initiative. This information is evidence-based research on the comparative effectiveness of prescription drugs in the same drug class. One of the best websites is <u>www.Oregonrx.org.</u> This website gives very specific information about the clinical trials, (including who sponsored them) and then gives a summary of

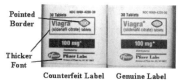

Counterfeit Label   Genuine Label

New genuine Viagra packaging with color-shift logo

It Could Happen To You
Many Americans have had to deal with the ramifications of counter-feit drugs distributed right here in the U.S. One such person was a seventeen-year-old male, suffering from anemia after undergoing a liver transplant, who was required to inject Epogen for treatment. He would wake up "screaming in agony" at night without knowing why. In the spring of 2002, his local pharmacy called the family and informed them that his last prescription refill was part of a counter-feit batch and that the young man had been injecting a counterfeit Epogen. When his family took the Epogen vial back to the pharma-cy, they found it to be very similar to the real thing, except that the *degree sign* on the vial was missing.[10]

CAUTION: CONSUMERS SHOULD DO ALL THEY CAN TO PROTECT THEMSELVES AND THEIR FAMILIES FROM COUNTERFEIT DRUGS. Be observant about the appearance of medications and their packaging. Also, read all the safety informa-tion in this chapter and check the author's website: www.prescription-pathway.com on a regular basis for up-to-date information.

Counterfeit Illustrations

Samples of the differences in counterfeit packaging and pills are illustrated below- Source:GAO report

Consumer Information

Consumer information available on safety and counterfeiting that readers should consider obtaining includes:

1. FDA Consumer Newsletter: For a sample copy of *FDA Consumer* and a subscription order form, write to: Food & Drug Administration, HFI-40, Rockville, MD. 20857.

2. U.S. General Services Administration Federal Citizen Information Center: Provides free or low-cost booklets on many consumer products including approximately 11 booklets related to drug products. Log on to: www.pueblo.gsa.gov to request a consumer information catalog.

3. Brochure: The information at the beginning of this chapter, "Your Medicine: Play It Safe" is available in a 12 page booklet in English and Spanish and includes a detachable, pocket-sized medication card. You can request a brochure at: www.ahrq.gov/consumer/safemeds/safemeds.htm.

4. "Talk about Prescriptions" (TAP PAK) from the National Council on Patient Information and Education (NCPIE). NCPIE is a great source for consumer drug safety information and their TAP PAK includes several brochures on how to recognize and respond to medication side effects, how to use OTC medications, etc. The TAP PAK can be ordered (no charge) from their website at www.talkaboutrx.org.

5. Public Citizen books and web site: As discussed earlier in the chapter, Public Citizen, a non-profit organization, has many great resources including the book: *"Worst Pill, Best Pill."* Check out their two websites at: www.citizen.org or www.worstpills.org.

6. MedlinePlus®: MedlinePlus® is service of the U.S. National Library of Medicine and the National Institutes of Health. It is a great source of drug information, directories, and health topics.

7. Author's website: www.prescriptionpathway.com. The author will continue to post any new information concerning specific counterfeit cases on this website.

Conclusion

Even with all the pharmaceutical system's safety problems and the increase in counterfeiting cases, most Americans remain confident in the FDA's ability to ensure that prescription drugs are safe. However, if the number of counterfeit cases continues to rise, consumers will lose their confidence. Drug safety has received so much media attention in the last couple of years, especially after the VIOXX scandal. The FDA has reacted (but maybe also *overacted*) by initiating many new safety measures. Some of the measures may work or some may just serve to slow the drug approval process down. Consumers and patients need to be ever vigilant to ensure the safety of the drug products they are taking. The best offense is for consumers and patients to be *active* members of their healthcare team and to keep informed as much as possible.

Read the information in this book. Talk to doctors, pharmacists, and other health care professionals. Read about any new counterfeit or tampered products from newspapers and websites and check out the website www.prescriptionpathway.com on a regular basis. Information is always the best defense.

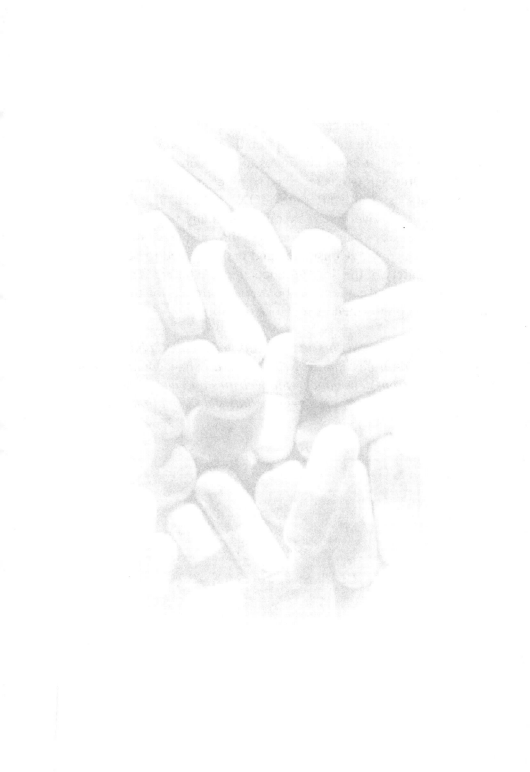

Chapter 4

Generics: The Best Buy

Introduction

Please! Call them something besides "generics!"

It's this author's theory that part of the problem with reassuring Americans that generic drugs are equal in quality to brand name drugs is due to their very name: *generics*. This term was coined in 1967 to describe a drug product that did not have a brand name or trademark. However, just the word itself conjures up images of inferior products. Most of the time, when consumers think of generic brands, they think of those bright yellow boxes on grocery store shelves. In addition, some generic food and cosmetic products (e.g. hand cream or crumbly generic-brand saltine crackers) are in fact substandard, which then leads to the argument that *all* generic products are inferior. However, this is not true with FDA approved generic drugs.   FDA-APPROVED GENERIC DRUG PRODUCTS ARE OF EQUAL QUALITY TO BRAND NAME DRUGS!

GENERICS ARE THE BEST WAY BY FAR TO SAVE MONEY ON PRESCRIPTION DRUGS WITHOUT SACRIFICING SAFETY OR EFFICACY.

Huge Savings

Generic drugs are equivalent to brand name drug products in terms of quality and performance, but they save consumers 70-80%! According to the National Association of Chain Drug Stores, in 2004, the average price of a generic prescription drug was $28.74. The average price of a prescription dispensed with a brand name drug was $96.02. That's an average savings of 70%!

Of the approximately 15,000 prescription drugs available today, over 7,000 of them have generic equivalents. According to the Congressional Budget office, generic drugs save consumers **$10 billion** a year at retail pharmacies. Additional billions can be saved when *hospitals* use generics. One well-known study estimated that for every 1% increase in the utilization of generic drugs, there is a corresponding $1.16 billion dollars in savings in health care dollars.[1] U.S. consumers could save nearly $9 billion a year with an increased use of generics.

Happily, the *use* of generics is increasing. Generic prescriptions as a percent of total prescriptions have increased from just 19% in 1984 to over 43% in 2003 and have a faster growth rate than brand name drugs. This was partly due to the decrease in development time for new active substances (brand name drugs) and partly due to the increased marketing of generics.

In 2004, the FDA approved 474 generics (note: this isn't 474 different drugs, but 400 different generic versions).

However, here is the kicker: ALTHOUGH 43% OF ALL PRESCRIPTIONS FILLED ARE GENERIC, GENERICS ACCOUNTED FOR LESS THAN 10% OF THE PHARMACEUTICAL DOLLAR SALES IN 2004! In other words, for every $1 spent on prescription drugs, only *10 cents* is spent on generics and *90 cents* spent on brand name drugs. The whole U.S. generic market it estimated at just $20 billion. Compare that to the sales of the top selling *brand* name drug ($6.3 billion for just 1 drug!) This further emphasizes the cost spread between generic and brand name prescription drugs. N*one* of the drugs in the top 50 prescription drugs by SALES were a generic formulation.

However, here is some good news for Americans: in the next 5 years, 67 major drugs are set to lose patent and/or exclusivity protection. In 2006-2007, $50 billion worth of brand name drugs are slated to come off patents. Hopefully, many of these drugs will be available in generic formulations.

The rule of thumb is that prices on the patented brand name drugs drop 20% in the first six months after a generic is approved for marketing, during which time only a single manufacturer has a 180-day exclusivity to sell a generic. However, now that consumers are more aware of the safety of generics, and healthcare plans continue to educate members to use generics, a drug can now lose 80-90% of its market share in just a few weeks. For example, Paxil, a brand name antidepressant, had a first-time generic competitor in September 2003. In August 2003, The Paxil brand had 100% of market share- by October 2003; it only had about 25% of the market.

Savings are huge when a generic makes it to market- consider that back in 2002 when Prozac first came open to generic competition, the price for a 20 mg. pill decreased from $3.13 per pill to just $2.10 a pill. Then, once the market had more than one generic manufacturer for Prozac, price dropped even more. By 2004, consumers could purchase a generic Prozac at Costco for less than 24 cents per pill! Generic competition always results in cost savings to the individual patient, as well as to the bottom line of U.S. total health care expenditures, *without compromising quality or safety.*

Generic Substitution

Most consumers don't realize that *if* there is a generic equivalent available for the prescription drug prescribed by their physician, they are usually receiving generics automatically. The major reason is that many states have passed laws requiring automatic generic substitutions if generics are available and equivalent. Currently, a total of 39 states permit substitution of generic products while 11 states mandate generic substitution.[2] Even if there isn't a law in a particular state, a physician can still write for a generic by signing on the right hand side of the prescription form indicating that substitution is permissible. In addition, most HMOs and other health insurance plans require generic substitutions.

(Some health plans report a 90% generic substitution rate for drugs with a generic equivalent.) However, a physician is always free to make a personal choice for each patient and can still prescribe a "brand name drug only," by signing for it on the *left* side of the prescription form. In these instances, the HMO or other health insurance company may still require the patient to pay a higher copay or the cost difference between the generic and brand name drug.

Generic Drugs and Bioequivalency

Definitions

So what exactly is a generic drug? By law, generic drug products evaluated by the FDA can be said to be "bioequivalent" to the original brand name drug, if it delivers the same amount of active ingredient(s) into the patient's bloodstream in the same amount of time.

One way scientists measure bioequivalence is to measure the time it takes the generic drug to reach the bloodstream and its concentration in the bloodstream in 36 healthy, normal volunteers. This gives scientists the rate and extent of absorption of the generic drug so that they can compare it to the original brand name drug.

The FDA has established a coding system to determine if a particular generic is equivalent. It assigns an "AB" rating if the generic product is considered to be therapeutically equivalent to a brand product when the testing done by the generic manufacturer demonstrates the brand and generic are bioequivalent.[3]

How the Generic versions receive FDA approval

There are 8 major parts to the FDA's review of a firm's application to a generic drug:[4]

- There must be an FDA approved brand name drug that is the reference for the proposed generic. The generic must have the same active ingredient or ingredients and the same labeled strength as the reference product. It must have the same dosage form (e.g. tablets, patches, liquids). It must be administered the same way (e.g. swallowed or by injection).

- The manufacturer must show that the generic drug is "bioequivalent" (see above.)
- The generic drug's labeling must be essentially the same as that of the approved drug.
- The firm must fully document the generic drug's chemistry, manufacturing steps and quality control measures. It must meets the same batch-to-batch requirements for strength, purity and quality and;
- The firm must assure the FDA that the raw materials and the finished product meet USP specifications.
- The firm must show that its generic drug maintains stability and the firm must monitor stability.
- The firm must provide a full description of the facilities it uses to manufacture, process, test, and package label and control the drug. It must certify that it complies with federal regulations about current good manufacturing practices and undergo an FDA inspection of the manufacturing facility to assure compliance (cGMP), as defined in the U.S. Code of Federal regulations.
- Before the FDA approves a generic drug, it usually conducts an inspection at the proposed manufacturing site to make sure the firm is capable of meeting its commitments, as well as assuring the product's consistency.

The Hatch-Waxman Act of 1984 created the framework for the more timely entry of generic drugs in the U.S. and assured FDA approval without compromising safety. The act streamlined the process, allowing generic drug companies to focus on proving that their drugs were equivalent, without requiring extensive clinical trials that would duplicate work already done by brand name companies. The Abbreviated New Drug Application (ANDA) used to approve generic drugs was born as a result of this legislation.

To obtain FDA approval, generic drug companies must:

1. Meet all the 8 requirements listed above.

2. File the ANDA. The ANDA process requires only information to show bioequivalence. This means that they must show the generic delivers the same amount of active ingredient in the same timeframe as the brand product. Rigorous bioequivalency testing must show that they meet specifications and are equal in strength, quality, purity, and potency.

3. Each ANDA must be filed with 1 of the following 4 certifications to indicated that a generic version can be sold in the U.S. 1) the brand drug is not patented, 2) all patents have expired, 3) the generic will not be marketed until all patents expire and 4) all patents are not infringed or are invalid. Incidentally, Number 4 is the requirement that is causing so many of the delays. In the past, generic drug companies would start *lining up at the FDA's parking lot* sometimes weeks before the first eligible day when they could legally file the ANDA. The *firm represented in the parking lot with the lowest numbered stamp* would receive the all-important 180 days of market exclusivity. That process has been improved upon so that all companies that file that first eligible day can be part of a "shared exclusivity."

4. The generic drug manufacturer is not required to pay for the expensive R & D with costly clinical trials. Instead, they are allowed to use the clinical trials performed by the brand company to prove the drug's safety and efficacy.

5. The generic manufacturer must develop its own shape for the pills; change the color or taste, or use flavorings or preservatives to create a unique appearance. The reason for the differences in looks is that trademark laws in the U.S. do not allow a generic drug to look exactly like brand name drugs already on the market. However, these ingredients must not affect the performance or effectiveness of the drug.

Consumers should know that there *must* be the potential of a substantial profit to be made by a generic manufacturer before it will embark on manufacturing a generic drug, which will require fighting all the patent and exclusivity arrangements, as well as injunctions and lawsuits, by the brand name companies. Just about any blockbuster drug (over $1 billion in sales a year) is going to warrant a financial investment for a generic version.

New kinds of generics

1. Authorized generics: Authorized generics are products *manufactured* by the innovator pharmaceutical company but *marketed without a brand name* through a generic company. The marketing company pays royalties to the brand company. Authorized generics are less expensive than the brand, but still more expensive than a regular generic. The authorized generic process once again demonstrates the fine line between brands and generics, with the only difference being the cost of the drug product to the consumer. Authorized generics are usually launched on or before the first day of another generic firm's 180-day marketing exclusivity. They are another way that brand name companies continue to maintain their market share (by receiving revenues for both brand and generic versions). The *generic drug industry* believes that authorized generics are taking unfair advantage of a loophole in the Hatch-Waxman legislation. However, the practice doesn't appear to break any laws and continues to be supported by the Courts, as well as the FDA. In 2005, there were approximately 21 authorized generics on the market (the practice began several years earlier.) In the future, consumers can expect to see more of them, as well as *multiple* authorized generics of the *same* drug.

2. Branded generics: This is a controversial new drug category that is a hybrid of brand name drugs and generics. Unlike regular generics, they are not biologically equivalent to the original brand name drugs and often have a slightly different formulation. The

drug is intended to act the same way in the body, but because it's not an exact match, it doesn't infringe on existing patents. (One example of a branded generic is the popular oral contraceptive Levora). Through an alternative method of drug approval, called 505 (b)(2), more than 100 applications for different dosage forms for existing brands have been approved in the forms like patches, alternate strengths and even switches of prescription drugs to over-the-counter drugs. This has been known as a "back door" process because it does not require the original proof of safety and effectiveness mandatory for approving new brand name drugs, nor does it require the same reams of data required to approve non-branded generics.[5] How this will work and what exactly will be the impact of this generic alternative is still unclear, since branded generics cannot be substituted in the pharmacy like other generics. It's also unclear how substantial the savings will turn out to be for the average consumer. Many generic manufacturers believe that allowing branded generics, especially during the all-important 180-day exclusivity period, will provide a strong disincentive for generic manufacturing and will keep prices artificially higher for longer periods of time. This same concern also applies to the authorized generics.

Safety of Generic Drugs

There was a time, maybe a decade ago, that generics were believed to be inferior. THAT IS NO LONGER THE CASE.

Over the past few years, there have been no newsworthy cases where there was a difference in the generic and brand name in regards to the rates of adverse events, as long as the generic purchased was a *U.S. FDA approved generic that had not been subject to tampering or counterfeiting*. However, consumers should be aware that sometimes the FDA lags behind in its on-site manufacturing reviews and is occasionally slow in taking a drug off the market (generic *or* brand). A good example is the antidepressant drug Serzone, which has already been taken off the market in Europe. Bristol-Myers Squibb, the brand name drug company, has stopped marketing the drug due to cases of severe liver toxicity. However, generic versions of the drug are still available in the U.S. (as of 2004), because the FDA has not chosen to require the removal of the drug from the market.

Generic substitutions for *biotechnology drugs* will continue to lag behind in generic substitutions. This is due to the fact that biotech companies maintain that most biotech drugs, such as interferons, growth hormones and proteins, do not lend themselves to generic production because living cell cultures yield considerable variation among batches. Consequently, biotech products require more testing than conventional drugs to ensure uniformity, potency, and purity. This also means it will cost more for companies to create generic versions. However, the *science* to fashion a generic biologics program is there; the FDA just needs to figure out how to implement a program for therapeutic equivalence. Experts believe that the biotech companies will be the first to create biotech generics, rather than the generic companies.

The FDA publishes a book called the "Orange Book" that lists all the generic medications that have been reviewed and are considered safe and bioequivalent. The FDA also assigns a rating for each generic. Consumers can search for generic equivalents by using the "Electronic Orange Book" at http://www.fda.gov/cder/ob/default.htm and search by proprietary "brand name," then search again by using the active ingredient name. The generic drug manufacturers are listed beside the "brand name" manufacturer when searching by the "active ingredient." In addition, readers can refer to Appendix B in this book for the Top 50 Most Prescribed Generic Alternatives.

When generic drugs are not bioequivalent

Over the last few years, an increasingly popular method used to decrease the costs of prescription drugs is to *replace* an expensive brand name drug for a generic that is <u>not</u> bioequivalent, but yet is in the same therapeutic class. This is being done based on the findings of what is known as evidence-based medicine and was discussed briefly in Chapter 2. - For example, a generic version of Mevacor has been recommended over Lipitor. Readers can find reviews of all the cholesterol-lowering drugs as well as up to 25 additional classes of drugs at www.oregonrx.com.

U.S. generics vs. drugs purchased from Canada

U.S. generics are almost always *less expensive* than Canadian generics. In fact, overall, *generic* drug prices in Canada are as much as 70% higher than those in the U.S.! This is due to many factors, including the drug pricing systems/procedures in Canada that leave little room for competition among generic drug companies (e.g., there are no price controls for Canadian generics). In fact, there are reports of Canadians crossing the U.S. border to buy their generics in the U.S.!

However, Americans still buy *brand name* prescription drugs in Canada because some may cost up to 40% less that their counterparts here in the U.S. For more information on purchasing prescription drugs in Canada, see *Chapter 13.*

Generics made by other countries

There is expected to be a marked rise in the number of foreign generics and foreign generic firms in 2006 and 2007, especially in India, Latin America, and China. This will continue to put added pricing pressures on U.S. generic companies and will affect what drugs will be imported from Europe via the Internet. Increasingly drug manufacturing is becoming more of a global industry.

Common misconceptions about generic drugs

There are many misconceptions about generic drugs including:
1. They are cheaper- therefore, they must be inferior. In a recent survey conducted by the pharmacy benefits company Medco Health

Solutions, only 47% of survey respondents state they would use generics to treat heart disease and only 56% said they would use generics to treat asthma, and 52% to treat diabetes. However, 79% would use generics to treat minor conditions like colds and flu.[6] This is probably the greatest misconception about generics-that they are inferior. Mark McClellan, who at the time was the FDA commissioner, was quoted as saying: "The FDA must do more than ever to help Americans get access to generic drugs, because they are as safe and effective as the brand name, while much less expensive."

2. Respected pharmaceutical companies produce brand name drugs but generics are only produced by second-rate companies. Again, not true. In fact, the same manufacturers who make brand name drugs make 75% of the generic drugs sold today! If consumers trust the brand name firms for the quality of their *brand name* drugs, why wouldn't they trust those same companies for their generic products? Ironically, the pharmaceutical industry has done a good job over the years of convincing the average American that their brand name drugs are superior. Now, they are in the same business! Big Pharma companies who also manufacture *generic* drugs include: Novartis, Merck, Pfizer, and Schering- Plough. For example, Novartis makes a generic version of AstraZeneca's Prilosec, which in turn has an over-the-counter version as well as a prescription version. The lines have blurred so much between class types (e.g. brand, generic, authorized generic) that the old misconceptions about generics no longer apply.

Speeding up the availability of generics- aided by the FDA and Congress

Both the FDA and Congress are working to streamline procedures and aid in the availability of generics *sooner* rather than later. Efforts include:

1. Drafting meaningful bioequivalent comparisons for "difficult to

manufacture" generic therapeutics, such as dermatological and inhaled products, as well as estrogen products and liposomal drugs that target therapy to selected tissues. (Currently, estrogen products sold today are derived from the urine of pregnant horses and many argue that this is not a bio-identical hormone. The FDA is looking at other options). Also, Pfizer is currently developing a non-hormonal drug to treat symptoms of menopause.

2. Developing policies regarding biologics- new biologics are among the most costly drugs.

3. Improving the efficiency and speed of generic approval and reducing the back-and forth between companies and the FDA. In recent years, 93% of ANDAs were not approved on the first review. Each cycle can mean months of delays.

4. Approving legislation that would close many of the loopholes in the Hatch-Waxman Act. First up, legislation was passed to allow only one automatic 30-month patent extension when a brand name pharmaceutical company challenges a generic filing. Next up: proposed legislation on Capitol Hill to eliminate that one remaining automatic 30-month stay and allow the courts to determine whether the brand company is entitled to a "preliminary injunction".

5. Cracking down on anticompetitive practices. This practice is probably the primary reason that Americans don't have access to affordable generics.

It Could Happen To You

<u>Always</u> ask if the drug you are purchasing at the pharmacy is a generic and always pay attention. <u>Don't</u> <u>assume</u> that you will receive a less costly generic, even if it is allowed or required by the State pharmacy laws. For example, a consumer we'll call Jane Doe was once filling a prescription for an antibiotic at a local drugstore and when it was time to check out, she was told to pay a *$30* copay. When she asked if the drug was a generic, the pharmacist told Jane that the generic version was out of stock so they were automatically filling the order with a brand name drug (and the copay was 3 times as much!) Instead, Jane Doe asked the pharmacist to provide just 2 or 3 pills right away and then asked the pharmacist to order a new supply of the generic version. Jane was then able to pay just $10 (instead of $30) by returning to the pharmacy the next day for the rest of the order.

Examples like the one above happen frequently. A new Consumer Reports Survey reported that 40% of their readers stated their drug-store was out of the medicine they needed at least once during the past year.[7]

Price comparison

The Table below shows just how inexpensive generics really are compared to their brand name counterpart for 15 popular prescription drugs:

Drug/Dosage----Brand 30Day Supply- (generic)	Generic $	Brand $	% Savings
1. Prilosec 10 mg (omeprazole)	32.99	117.59	72%
2. Mevacor 20 mg (lovastatin)	19.49	67.69	71%
3. Zovirax 200 mg (acyclovir)	11.07	53.19	79%
4. Prozac 20 mg. (fluoxetine)	6.59	31.99	79%
5. Retina-A. .45 mg tube (tretinoin)	54.19	88.49	38%
6. Glucophage-500 mg	7.09	22.69	69%
7. Glucotrol XL 10 mg	17.69	27.19	35%
8. Synthroid 100 mcg (Levothyroxine)	10.09	16.09	33%
9. Lasix 20 mg (furosemide)	4.39	8.99	51%
10. Keflex 250 mg. (cephalexin)	7.49	52.29	86%
11. Paxil 20 mg (paroxetine)	22.69	84.69	73%
12. Tenormin 50 mg. (atenolol)	11.37	63.47	80%
13. Lopressor 100 mg (metroprolol)	7.59	48.59	84%
14. Naprosyn 250 mg. (Naproxen)	6.99	34.09	79%
15. Ventolin 90 mcg. Inhaler (albuterol)	6.29	38.29	84%

Consumer information

Excellent sources of consumer information regarding generic drugs are available from both the FDA and the Generic Pharmaceutical Association (GPHA).

Recommended publications include:

FDA: DHHS Publication No. 02-3242, www.fda.gov-   Brochure: "You know the questions that go through your mind when you take your generic drug? Here are the answers."
GPHA website: See www.gpha.com for more information.

Conclusion

President George W. Bush was quoted in February 2003 as saying: "...By saving consumers billions of dollars in prescription drug costs, generic drugs play a critical role in helping ensure that all American's have access to lifesaving drugs and advancements in medicine to help them live better and longer lives". This is one message he's given to consumers that they should take to heart.

An argument could even be made that taking a generic medication may in fact be safer. One reason is that most of the serious side effects found in prescription drugs are usually discovered in the first few years a drug is on the market, (if they're not found during clinical trials). A study, led by Dr. Karen Lasser of Cambridge Hospital and Harvard Medical School, found that of the 548 drugs approved from 1975 through 1999, 56 (or more than 10%) were later given a serious side effect warning or taken off the market for safety reasons.[8]   Remember all the hubbub surrounding fen-phen, the diet drug? So many people died from heart failure due to fen-phen that the FDA finally took it off the market. While this theory is not completely based on scientific fact, it's definitely something to consider.

Another thought worth considering: Counterfeiters rarely tamper with generic drugs- there isn't enough profit in it.

APPENDIX B contains a cross reference of 50 of the most common generic prescription drugs prescribed, as well as the name of their brand name counterparts. Readers should use this list to ensure that they are receiving the generic version of prescribed drugs whenever possible. In addition, readers can check the author's website: www.prescriptionpathway.com for updates on new generic versions of popular brand name prescription drugs. The website also contains recent information of any prescription drug withdrawals, both generic *and* brand.

Chapter 5

Pharmaceutical Companies- Friend or Foe

> TIP: Get something free from the pharmaceutical companies!
> Ask your physician for drug samples, if the drug being prescribed is a
> brand name drug and not covered by your insurance. Also, check out
> the drug company's websites for coupons for free 7- day trials.

Introduction

The pharmaceutical industry consists of a cadre of Fortune 500 companies, all with shareholders and Wall Street expectations for double-digit profits. For instance, in 2002, the pharmaceutical company who manufactures the #1 prescription drug in America reported profits of $9.1 billion on revenues of $32.4 billion (28%). Compare this to General Electric and you see that the drug company's profit is more than 2 times as great, - Wal-Mart -9 times as great and, gasp, greater than General Motors by 31 times![1] The combination of huge profits, media notoriety, and gigantic political clout has caused these multinational pharmaceutical giants to be referred by many as "Big Pharma." When the 10 largest pharmaceutical corporations can account for almost 60% of total U.S. prescription drug sales, it's easy to see why the name might be well deserved.

Many believe that the U.S. pharmaceutical industry is a double-edged sword. On the one hand, the industry helped provide financial support for the U.S. during the fallout of American prosperity after 9/11. The profitability of this industry helped prop up the American economy with double digit profits. On the other hand, retail prices of prescription drugs (especially brand name drugs) had been priced beyond what the average American could afford in a recovering economy- or any economy- and the prices just keep escalating. In addition, private individuals who are uninsured, including seniors and low-income families, are the ones who pay the highest retail prescription prices. This in fact is a major area where the U.S. differs from other developed countries. America has many different prices for many different groups of people, with the highest prices being paid by those with the lowest income. In other countries, the price is the same, or even less for the low-income population (e.g. India- where the poor receive drugs at cost price).

For those not working in the drug industry, there are many unanswered questions. Americans want to know "<u>why</u>." Why do drugs cost so much? Why are pharmaceutical companies price gouging, or are they? Why has the pharmaceutical industry been called the "eight-hundred-pound gorilla" (as quoted by Dr. Marcia Angell in her book: *"The Truth about the Drug Companies*)? Are the pharmaceutical companies the reason that Americans can't legally buy prescription drugs in Canada? Can they really be that greedy?

The purpose of this chapter is to attempt to present an objective point of view of the pharmaceutical industry. However, some of the author's biases will still be self-evident, based on personal knowledge and the experience from working inside the industry as a pharmaceutical sales representative ("detail rep") and from dealing with Big Pharma for the past thirty years.

To begin, let's discuss a few plain simple truths about pharmaceutical companies:

- The 16 giant pharmaceutical companies, (Big Pharma), produce socially beneficial products that *improve the lives of billions of people.* However, first and foremost they are profit-making businesses with Boards and Investors. Although their end products are altruistic, these for-profit businesses still have a bottom line and must make a healthy profit for their shareholders.

- The 16 giant pharmaceutical companies have a goal to launch two new products per year. In 2002, this target had been achieved by only 2 of the 16 companies. In 2003, 33% of the companies had not launched a single new product in the U.S.!

- Companies appear to be spending more and more resources on developing further indications and line extensions (e.g. an extended release form) to their *existing* blockbuster products in order to enhance their return on R & D investment, rather than developing new innovative products.

- According to Fortune 500 Magazine, the pharmaceutical industry was the 3rd most profitable industry in the U.S. in 2003 and more than 3 times as profitable as the median for all Fortune 500 companies.[2] From 1995-2002, they were the number 1 most profitable industry.

- All the new brand name pharmaceutical products created by Big Pharma achieve up to 85% of their sales in the U.S., In other words, Big Pharma companies receive most of their profits from Americans, even when their products are manufactured and sold worldwide.[3]

In order to understand how the pharmaceutical companies' business practices effect consumers' pocketbooks, and to understand both sides of the drug "coin", this chapter is divided into two parts: "the foe and the friend".

The "Foe"- why the bad rap?

A Harris poll published in June 2004 asked Americans "Do you think pharmaceutical and drug companies generally do a good job of service to their consumers?" In 1997, 79% answered yes; however in 2004, only 44% said yes, placing them only slightly above oil companies (32%) and tobacco companies (30%). A larger portion surveyed thought they were doing a bad job (48%).[4]

Many Americans blame Big Pharma for the rising costs of prescription drugs. It's easy to see why, when the more transparent some of the pharmaceutical industry practices become, the more concerned consumers are.

And costs *do* keep rising at rates much higher than inflation, with some studies estimating it to be 7-8% overall. A survey conducted by AARP in 2005 showed that wholesale prices for popular brand name drugs increased an average of 7.1%, more than twice the general inflation rate. Since the end of 1999, 153 brand name drugs raised prices an average of 35%![5] On top of that, many of the pharmaceutical companies raised their prices on brand name drugs in *early 2005*, right *after* the presidential election and *before* negotiating discounts with Medicare pharmacy intermediaries. This implies that that the "20%" discount that will be reported to the public or in the media for the Medicare prescription benefit, will really only be 10-15% off of 2004 prices. The pharmaceutical industry is estimated to make an additional *$50 billion* or more in revenue with the new Medicare benefit.

Examples of Alleged Abuses by Big Pharma:

Alleged abuses by Big Pharma that have occurred over the past few years, include:

1. In 2001, a pharmaceutical company "pleaded guilty to conspiring with doctors in a scheme to overcharge government insurance programs for reimbursement for its prostate cancer drug Lupron."[6]

2. Neurontin- Currently, this drug is approved by the FDA *only* for the treatment of epilepsy. However, it became a 2.5 billion a year blockbuster drug the last few years because it was illegally marketed by the company for attention deficit disorder, migraine, and bipolar disease- (see the off-label paragraph later in this chapter).

3. New York City filed a lawsuit against 44 pharmaceutical companies, alleging overcharging of Medicaid by artificially inflating the average wholesale prices (AWPs.) (The case is still pending.) Illinois followed in 2005 with a similar lawsuit. AWPs are the prices manufacturers use to sell drugs to their customers e.g. physicians, pharmacies and HMOs. In the healthcare business, "AWP" has been called "Ain't Whatcha Paid" because in reality, almost no one pays AWP.

4. Deficiencies found in manufacturing plants have resulted in hundreds of millions of fines. Plants and sites with manufacturing problems have been identified in Puerto Rico and other sites. Recently, the FDA raided one of the Big Pharma plants in Puerto Rico and confiscated all of its prescription drugs for specific batches of an antidepressant and a diabetes agent. It turns out the antidepressant tablets could split apart and the diabetes agent tablets did not have an accurate dose of its active ingredient.

5. Big Pharma has been accused of hiding negative information about clinical trials (see Chapter 2.) One example includes several companies who allegedly suppressed evidence of increased suicide risks in children taking antidepressants. Another recent example that played out in public is the huge VIOXX /COX-2 inhibitors scandal that alleges Merck *knew* about the increased risk of cardiac events as early as 1996, but hid the information from both federal regulators and consumers.

6. Some pharmaceutical companies, according to the Federal Trade Commission, have allegedly made deals with generic firms to delay the sale of generic versions of their brand name drugs. However, in early 2005, one state court upheld a ruling that this practice was not illegal. This will continue to have far reaching implications as Americans and patient advocates strive to increase the number of available generic drugs.

7. Some companies have been accused of using sales incentives to get wholesalers to overstock their shelves, thus driving up revenue and helping the drug companies meet sales targets.

*Please note: the above instances are *alleged* abuses and may or not have been proven to be correct. What *is* certain, however, is that the pharmaceutical industry's image has been tarnished over the past few years by numerous allegations such as these and there seems no reason to believe the industry can improve their image anytime soon. Big Pharma will have to do more than show a few glossy TV ads touting all the good they accomplish in order to convince Americans that they are not being ripped off.

Cost of R & D is <u>less</u> than marketing and sales costs

The reason cited most often by Big Pharma for the high cost of prescription drugs is the cost of <u>research and development</u> (R & D.) It is true that pharmaceutical companies *are* one of a handful of company types that spend a disproportionate amount of their revenues on R & D.

But what bothers most consumers is that according to some experts, the marketing and promotion costs are **double** that of R& D costs! For example, one of the major pharmaceutical companies poured nearly <u>$500 million</u> in the first year on promotion of one brand name drug.[6] According to some experts, $500 million could pay for the R & D for 1-2 brand new drugs!

The average prescription cost was $63.59 in 2004. Of that amount, it is estimated that only *12% was spent on R & D while 2 ½ times* as much (or 26%) was spent on sales, marketing, and administration! According to an academic study by the Stanford University Center for Research in Disease Prevention, the pharmaceutical industry spent a whopping *$12.7 billion* in sales, marketing, and advertising in 2003. However, the $12+ billion may be a conservative estimate. When searching for the truth, it is difficult to obtain the facts on how much is really spent on R & D and how much is spent on marketing. According to *PhRMA,* the pharmaceutical companies' trade organization, (member) drug companies spent $38.8 billion on R & D industry-wide in 2004 ($30.6 billion was spent domestically and 8.2 billion abroad.) [7] This $38.8 billion may seem to be a "WOW," until you look at the total picture, where sales revenue for the same period was over $217 billion! However, what the public can't confirm is what's actually calculated by Big Pharma as R & D expenses. In fact, no one has actually seen any of the Big Pharma financial statements. The U.S. GAO (General Accounting Office) tried unsuccessfully for years to obtain government approval to look at the Big Pharma's financials until eventually they just gave up. According to a GAO report in February 2003, "Pharma have been overstating their R & D costs by 60% for years." Included in that R & D number is what's known as "opportunity costs," which is money that would have been made by the drug developer if the R & D funds had been invested in *equities* instead of R & D. There is also the legitimate argument that much of the R & D is already paid for by government programs such as the National Institutes of Health (NIH). In fact, NIH spends over $23 billion every year on drug research. According to Dr. Bernadine Healy, a former NIH director, "there's no other industry in which you have so much public investment in the fundamental knowledge that enables......the development of the commercial industry itself." Compare this government investment to other industries (for example, the airline industry). The airlines would love to have their business underwritten by the government; especially in the aftermath of 9/11, when some of the companies are unable to get sufficient government loans to stay in business.

A powerful lobbying group

The pharmaceutical industry employs at least 526 Washington lobbyists. *This means there are at least a hundred more registered lobbyists than there are members of Congress!* The drug companies spent a record $158 million on lobbying activities in 2004 and $17 million more in 2004 political campaign contributions (67% to Republicans.)[8] In fact, PhRMA spent more on lobbying than any other sector from 1999-2001.[9] An example of how ridiculous this has become was demonstrated after 500 lobbyists descended on the Capitol in the state of Maine at a time when controversial pharmaceutical legislation was recommended, but challenged for three years all the way to the U.S. Supreme Court. The new legislation required drug companies to negotiate big discounts to *all uninsured* residents with incomes up to 350% of the federal poverty level and not just to Medicaid recipients. It's easy to see why Big Pharma wouldn't like the idea of a legal mandate requiring that discounts be given to *everyone*-this would not only cut profits but would set a precedence. And although prescription sales in Maine account for only 1% of all total drug spending, many people in the pharmaceutical industry worried it would bring the U.S. one step closer to government price controls. However, despite heavy lobbying by Big Pharma, the legislation was upheld by the Supreme Court of Maine in 2003. Now in 2005, this is being played out once again in California.

Patents, exclusivity and other games

Ever since the Hatch-Waxman Act was passed in 1984 in order to "protect" the pharmaceutical companies from generic companies infringing on their patents, there have many abuses by the brand name drug companies. The patent and exclusivity issues have already been discussed in Chapter 2, but to emphasize the abuse of this legislation, one just has to read the quote by Senator Orrin Hatch, R-Utah who originally co-authored the all-important Hatch-Waxman Act: "The pharmaceutical companies under this law have looked for every loophole they could possibly find to keep generics off the market."

Another way the pharmaceutical companies have gamed the system is with the pediatric exclusivity regulations implemented in 1997. This measure provides incentives to the drug companies to conduct tests on children by granting an additional 6 months of exclusivity. As a consequence of the legislation, 332 new pediatric drug studies were begun within a 3-year period and a total of 100 drugs have received new pediatric labeling since 1998. The intent was to establish precise dosages and side effects for children, but the result has been an extension of brand name prices for drugs that may or may not have a generic equivalent. Senator Waxman, the other co-author of the bill has admitted: "The exclusivity clause had given the companies an unintended 'windfall' of billions of dollars at the expense of consumers who were denied six months of lower generic prices." One example of the "windfall" for just one large drug company that paid an estimated $2-$4 million on clinical trials for children on just *one* drug was an extra *$1.2 billion* in sales! Putting this into perspective, this amount is $1.2 billion more than the entire budget of the National Institute of Child Health and amounts to a 30,000-60,000% return on investment!

Another strategy that often brings billions in profits to Big Pharma is the prohibition of generic competition through litigation. If a "blockbuster" drug that generates up to $3 billion in sales is going off patent and the pharmaceutical company can delay a generic for 6 months or more, there is still a huge profit to be made, even after court costs.

The Amgen paradigm

A great example of how new breakthrough drugs are discovered, manufactured and distributed with very little R & D investment by the companies themselves, is found in the story of the biotech company: Amgen. The company that came to be known as *Amgen* manufactured the 1st biotech blockbuster drug called Epogen. This transformed a struggling start-up company into the largest and most profitable biotech company in the world in just a few years. The eventual product prevented tens of thousands of deaths from tainted blood transfusions and enabled millions of cancer and dialysis patients to live longer and more productive lives. It began with a biochemistry professor at University Chicago named Eugene Goldwasser. He spent 20 years doing research, *all paid for by the federal government*. He identified and purified the first small vial of human erythropoietin. After nearly two decades, he decided to work exclusively with Amgen, known then as Applied Molecular Genetics, to test the protein and to eventually manufacture a product that could be marketed. In 1981, this small company began sequencing the protein. In 1983, they filed an NDA and began conducting clinical trials. Just 3½ years later, they received FDA approval.

In other words, Amgen hit pay dirt. Professor Goldwasser spent twenty years testing the drug and struggling to obtain R & D funds. However, after only spending a few years in testing, (and an unknown amount of money, though it's thought to be in the millions, not billions), Amgen received a patent and has been making brand name type profits from this drug for the past 17 years. Amgen has made billions on this intellectual capital. In addition, Medicare is the primary payer. In other words, American tax dollars are being used to pay the Medicare bill; not for 20 years of R & D, but rather to line the pocket of the 1st biotech company who has reaped billions in profits. Although a percentage of the profits *are* going towards the development of new biotech drugs, a substantial portion is just pure profit. (Note: this Amgen commentary was taken from information in the excellent book: "*The 800 Million Dollar Pill*" by Merrill Goozner.) [10] On top of all this, Amgen has not developed any truly new significant products in a long time.

Unlawful or "gray area" marketing tactics

Marketing "off-label" uses

A big pharmaceutical scandal in 2004 involved the U.S.'s largest pharmaceutical company who was allegedly found to be marketing one of its blockbuster drugs for several "off-label" uses. Off-label describes the practice of prescribing a drug for diseases/conditions for which the drug does <u>not</u> have FDA approval. *IT IS ILLEGAL for pharmaceutical companies to promote and market a prescription drug for any indication <u>not</u> approved by the FDA.* (This particular case has since been settled and the drug company obliged to pay a $430 million settlement.) This is not an isolated incident either and is another example of an alleged abuse executed by pharmaceutical companies. An estimated 500 drugs are currently under fire in off-label marketing investigations. Company payouts in "whistle-blower" cases have grown from $500 million in 1999 to 1.7 billion in 2003.[11]

However, readers should be advised that it is <u>not</u> illegal for a physician to *prescribe* a drug for an off-label use <u>if</u> the physician believes the benefits of the drug will outweigh the risks (e.g. for cancer treatments). The greatest problems with prescribing these drugs for off-label use happen when physicians fail to inform their patients that the drug being prescribed has *not* been approved by the FDA for their particular condition. For more information on drugs being used for off-label medical conditions, readers can check out the U.S. Pharmacopeia's website at www. usp.org.

"Buying the Business" and other purported kickbacks"

It's been no secret that for decades, pharmaceutical companies have been accused of "buying the business" with extravagant gifts. These free gifts have included such things as resort weekends, dinners, and travel to conferences and sporting events. While this is a common practice by many corporations <u>not</u> involved in health care, patients understandably don't like the idea of physicians deciding their prescribing habits based on who gave them the most expensive gifts. Often the best drugs, with the best value, are generics for which _no_ advertising or marketing is done.

Some of the extravagances used to buy the business and influence prescribing habits were reined in during the late 1990s. This is partially due to the fact that the FDA created pharmaceutical marketing guidelines to limit the gifts to physicians. Since 1990, the American Medical Association has developed gift-giving guidelines under which doctors are _not_ supposed to accept anything worth more than $100. In addition, in April 2002, PhRMA announced a new code of conduct; the codes required that all marketing campaigns to physicians had to be educational. Pharmaceutical companies could only underwrite educational conferences, provide modest meals that accompanied informational presentations and reimburse doctors only as "consultants."[12] (There were more than 200,000 if these "educational meetings" in 2004.) In addition, the U.S. Health & Humans Services Department proposed new standards that could leave drug makers open to prosecution for fraud or kickbacks if they offered extravagant freebies.[13] However, even with so many guidelines, the practice of self-regulation apparently isn't working _entirely_ as abuses continue to be reported.

Many health care providers are tired of inappropriate marketing tactics. The drug industry spent _$22 billion_ last year marketing to doctors using more than _90,000_ sales reps.[14] It's gotten to the point that the sales reps outnumber the physicians! Additionally, sales calls are almost always geared to the most expensive brand name drugs. As cited in an article in USA today in 2004, many hospitals and clinics are now reviewing their policies of allowing pharmaceutical representatives to meet with their physicians. For example, the University of Wisconsin Hospital and Clinics has implemented a disciplinary program for drug representatives to follow. Drug company representatives with three violations to existing policies- (for offenses such as giving out food or loitering outside doctor's lounges) - might expect to lose their hospital access for 6 months.[15]

(See more in the "Tales of a pharmaceutical sales rep" later in this chapter).

More "subtle: manipulations

Besides the overt alleged abuses, there are more subtle manipulations at play. Many times, pharmaceutical companies *fund* the very clinical trials on which guidelines and standard practices of care are developed. This practice arguably creates a conflict of interest. One fairly recent example is the new National Institutes of Health guidelines created using five major studies (funded by the pharmaceutical companies) to substantiate claims than individuals can reduce LDL and cholesterol levels and thereby reduce the risk of heart disease by taking "statins". (Statins are cholesterol-lowering drugs like Lipitor, Zocor, and the new Zetia.) *Coincidentally*, the new guidelines were issued *just 2 weeks prior* to the launch of a new combination drug that combines Zetia and Zocor (called Vytorin.) The studies on which the guidelines are based show that Vytorin is more effective in lowering LDL. Incidentally, Vytorin, costs approximately **$2.63 a pill,** while an older, but still effective cholesterol-lowering agent, available in generic form, (lovastatin), costs only 92 cents or $1.31 a day.

Another strategy used by Big Pharma to keep their market share is to seek FDA approval for an OTC "switch." (This has happened in the cases of both Claritin and Prilosec.) Once a prescription drug goes off patent, the pharmaceutical company has the potential to lose huge profits to generic companies. However, if they can get approval to *switch the drug to OTC* status, they maintain a major portion of the market share. As succinctly written by Fran Hawthorne in her book, *The Merck Druggernaut*: "the manufacturer also figured that if they couldn't get a full dollar for a drug as a brand name prescription, it was better to pick up a nickel on an OTC sale than lose everything to a generic."[16] In the case of Claritin, this has definitely turned out to be true. The drug manufacturer has had more than $1 billion in U.S. sales since Claritin was granted OTC status. The drug remains among the top three OTC drugs sold in the U.S.

Choking off the drug supply to Canada

Many consumers are very angry that at least four of the giant pharmaceutical companies have begun "blacklisting" Canadian pharmacies that export medications into the U.S. They have threatened to choke off supplies of brand name drugs to Canadian wholesalers and distributors who sell to Americans through online pharmacies. This in turn might then jeopardize the prescription drug supply for Canadians. The drug companies say they are ensuring adequate supplies for Canadians and protecting the safety of the consumers. However, to the public, this just looks like strong-arm tactics and more evidence of Big Pharma's greed.

Direct To Consumer (DTC) Advertising

In 1997, the FDA issued new guidelines that relaxed the codes for broadcast ads. This changed the face of pharmaceutical advertising and the ubiquitous Direct to Consumer (DTC) ad was born. DTC ads for drugs appear on television and in print ads. (And yes, over and over and over again!) Take for example one small magazine, Readers Digest: in just one magazine in one month, there were 15 different OTC and prescription drug ads.[17]

Spending on DTC advertising soared from $2.4 billion in 2001 to **$4.1 billion** in 2004. Of that amount, $3.0 billion was spent on TV ads and $1.1 billion on print ads (this included only $5 million on the Internet, although this is expected to increase.) [18] Most DTC marketing is focused on what is known as "lifestyle ailments" such as allergies, arthritis, cholesterol, insomnia, obesity, and sexual dysfunction. Of course, the drugs marketed though DTC are _not_ inexpensive generics, but the rather new most expensive brand name drugs.

Schering-Plough's DTC marketing of _prescription_ Claritin in 1998 set the standard for what was to come. (Note: this is _prior_ to OTC status). The company paid out a then _unprecedented $136 million_ worldwide for advertising; but the gamble paid off: sales skyrocketed 35% to 3.5 billion!"

Ethical dilemmas are raised by advertising for medicines that affect people's health as opposed to advertising for shoes, clothes, or avocados. Only one other country in the world, New Zealand, allows DTC marketing, and even they are reviewing the practice. Critics say that the ads influence physician prescribing patterns and affect the physician-patient relationship, although an FDA survey showed that when patients asked for a prescription for a specific drug, the doctor's obliged only 57% of the time.[19] Also, the advertising then leads to an increase in sales of *expensive* prescription drugs, of which more than half are bought *not* by consumers but by the government (e.g. Medicare and Medicaid-with *tax payer's money),* and by employers.

The FDA is charged with the responsibility of monitoring the DTC ads for false and/or misleading advertising. Enforcement includes issuing warning letters as well as collecting fines. In 2003, the FDA collected over $800 million in fines from the pharmaceutical industry for misleading statements and non-compliance with the advertising regulations. What happens frequently however is that a broadcast ad may run for 6 months to a year *before* the drug company is told to revise it or to cease and desist. In general, *pharmaceutical companies* can never go wrong by having a patient say to his/her physician: "I'm having this problem, what can I do?"

As of 2004, there has been a shift by many of the drug companies to change their DTC ads to be more general, and to focus on a *disease* rather than on just one particular drug. They are running general ads as a type of "image repair." Although a particular drug or website may not be mentioned until the end of the commercial, many see this as just a smoke screen. There are only a few industries (tobacco, alcohol, and oil companies) whose public image is so tarnished that they need to spend billions of dollars just to improve it.

Now: the "Friend"

Development of drugs for cancer, AIDs, asthma and diabetes

When looking for the good that pharmaceutical companies do, at the top of the list is the creation of new drugs for cancer, AIDS, and other life threatening and chronic diseases. Drugs prolong life, create a better quality of life, and provide cures for symptoms, if not always for the underlying diseases. Often, they decrease the need for a more invasive treatment such as surgery. However, these great new advances in biotechnology and pharmacology come at a great cost. While the newer drugs have a better side effect profile and prolong life, the cost of these advances is staggering. Older chemotherapy drugs cost as little as $63 for an initial 8-week treatment. However, add a new drug like Avastin to standard chemotherapy and the price increases to $21,000. Add Erbitux, and the price increases to $31,000. These drugs can extend survival by 21 months or more. However, the cost of treating all 56,000 Americans with advanced colorectal cancer, for example, could total as much as $1.2 billion. Nevertheless, if it is you or your family with this disease, no price is too high.

Donations

Big Pharma has been known to donate prescription drugs in emergency and non-emergency circumstances. For example, Big Pharma donated medications after the devastating tsunami in December 2004. Merck, which has a reputation for more philanthropic deeds, donated supplies of Mectizan, a drug that helps control river blindness, to poor nations in Africa and Latin America in 1987.[20] Sadly; the *proportion* of their revenues that go to charitable causes as compared to many other American corporations is still relatively small.

99

Drug Samples

For years pharmaceutical companies have been providing physicians with samples of prescription and OTC drugs to distribute to their patients free of charge. In addition, drug samples (e.g. boxes containing a 14-30 day supply) have long been one of the best marketing tools used by the pharmaceutical industry. It's the primary method employed to sway physicians to prescribe newer, more expensive medications.

On the positive side, drug samples have the following benefits:
- Provides free access to medications.
- Creates an opportunity for a trial of the new medication in order to determine the benefits and risks of the medication in individual patients.
- Provides the physician with an opportunity to observe the effects of the drugs in his or her own patient population.[21]

On the negative side, problems with distributing drug samples include:
- Physicians often give the samples to friends and/or relatives rather than patients.
- Sample distribution takes the pharmacist out of the dispensing and patient-counseling process for at least the first 14-30 days.

Although drug samples do create problems, if a consumer doesn't have prescription drug coverage and the physician wants to prescribe a new expensive brand name drug for his patient, then drug samples can still be helpful. However, readers should know that the *samples might not always be available.* The only way to know is to ask the physician or other health practitioner during the office visit or telephone consultation.

Drug Coupons

Drug coupons are issued by the pharmaceutical companies as a marketing tool and are usually for a very short duration, e.g., 7 days of treatment.). More often that not, the coupons are for chronic medications guaranteeing the patient's commitment to long-term purchases. However, a coupon can still provide a 25% savings for a 1-month supply - it also gives the patient and the physician the opportunity to evaluate the drug's effectiveness and side effect profile. The major hindrance is that a patient has to have the coupon in hand *during* the physician office visit so that a prescription for the free 7-day supply can be obtained, as well as the prescription for a 30-90 supply. A few of the websites that offer coupons include: www.celebrex.com. www.lipitor.com, www.purplepill.com (Nexium), www.aricept.com, www.diflucan.com, www.viagra.com, www.zoloft.com, www.zyrtec.com and www.healthybp.com.

Patient Assistance Programs

Pharmaceutical companies <u>do</u> provide prescription drugs to low-income individuals through their Patient Assistance Programs (PAPs). See chapter <u>9</u> for detailed information on PAPs. Also, you can go to the PhRMA websites at www.healthypatients.org. or www.pparx.org for more information. An even better website can be found at: www.rxassist.org.

DTC advertising- it can be a "positive" too

There are some pros for permitting DTC advertising, which is why DTC ads are presented here under both the "friend" and the "foe" portion of this chapter. DTC ads may in fact empower patients and encourage physician-patient communication. One of the hardest things for many patients to do is to talk to their physicians and hold them accountable for their actions. DTC ads provide at least some information on drug therapy options so that patients can have that two-way dialogue with their physicians, nurses, and pharmacists. In this information age, patients want to be informed and they want to move towards more self-care. **Access + Knowledge= Power**.

A survey conducted by the National Consumer League in 2003 found:[22]
1. More than half of adults who saw an ad of interest were motivated to take action after seeing the ad (57% among all adults and 58% among seniors- this is equal to 12% of all adults and 13% of seniors).

2. Overall, those who spoke with their doctor about the medicine they saw advertised were very positive about how it impacted their discussion.
3. In the end, 71% of all adults and 72% of seniors who spoke with their doctor about an advertised medication say their doctor prescribed the medication and it helped their condition (this equals 4% of all adults and seniors). Note: this is a higher percentage than has been reported in other surveys (see below).

In another survey of 1,500 Americans by Rodale Inc, publisher of *Prevention* magazine, the following results were reported:[23]
1. 84% say prescription drug ads tell them about new treatments
2. 78% say the ads allow people to be more involved with their own medical care.
3. 34% say they have talked to their doctor about an advertised medicine and of those, 21% asked for a prescription.

The physicians seemed mixed in their reaction to DTC ads. One report showed that 40% of *physicians* believe the ads have a positive effect on their patients and practice, although 30% say the opposite and 30% see no effect at all .[24]

In conclusion, DTC advertising works and in general, most consumers were satisfied with the results of the drugs and appreciated the opportunity of having a two-way communication about the drugs they saw advertised.

Propping Up the Economy

One of life's realities is that the pharmaceutical and biotech companies continue to keep the economy humming with their financial success. With few exceptions, brand firms continue to post positive sales and revenue growth, often with double-digit returns. The double-digit profits are a curse for the average consumer who cannot afford a prescription that costs $9,600 a year, but the drug sector has been a boon to Wall Street investors and therefore, aids in a healthy economy. What happens on Wall Street is very dependent on what happens with the Fortune 500 companies. Over the past few years as the U.S. has struggled to recover from 9/11, terrorism, the war in Iraq, and the burst of the Internet bubble, the 16 drug companies, and 2 of the biotech companies that make up "Big Pharma" have continued to provide hope and security for the bottom line in business. This is both a blessing and a curse for the pharmaceutical industry and thus bears mention.

Globalization

Another significant fact is that the pharmaceutical industry is now a global one. Most of Big Pharma has manufacturing plants in other countries. While the FDA *does* monitor these plants, requirements for packaging and labeling for those that are sold in the U.S., and other countries may be different. More than **$70 billion** of our prescription drugs are manufactured and then "imported" into the U.S. by the drug manufacturers. Again the line blurs. Many Americans still think that all prescription drugs are manufactured right here in the U.S. In addition, there are also *generic* manufacturing plants located in other countries such as India. They must also comply with FDA guidelines in order to market and sell their drug products here. It is a confusing yet compelling global market.

Tales of a pharmaceutical sales rep

A physician once told the author of this book that the prescription drug manufactured by her mid-size pharmaceutical company (her employer) was probably a better drug than the drug he usually prescribed. However, the physician was honest in admitting that *when it came time to prescribe a blood pressure medication, he usually prescribed the drug made by the company that had sent him and his wife to Cancun, Mexico for a conference.* Somehow, whether conscious or subconscious, the extravagant gifts seem to instill an obligation. There was a survey conducted in 2000 by Scott-Levin that seems to

---

confirm this personal anecdote. In this study, more than half the physicians attending events at restaurants and hotels said they intended to begin or increase their prescriptions of the products that were promoted at those events. Consumers have to believe that pharmaceutical companies wouldn't continue these marketing techniques if they didn't have proof that they worked.

As a pharmaceutical sales representative for a *mid-sized* company, the author was required to obtain prior approval from the New Jersey home office for a $50 lunch. However, at that time in the early 1990's, there were other companies spending hundreds or thousands of dollars on lunches, coffee mug warmers, calculators and all matter of freebies. (There is a great term for these give-a-ways- "tchotchkes"-they do nothing to educate or help the patient, but rather keep product names visible to physicians at all times). Although this is very common and considered by many Fortune 500 companies to be an acceptable practice, the moral and ethical principles are definitely questionable, especially when the end result is increased drug prices. Some say that ethics are not a consideration, as long as it doesn't hurt the patients and as long as it's legal; however, many disagree. Does your doctor really need another coffee mug warmer?

Another "detail rep" story: For better or worse, there is also the perception that pharmaceutical representatives are just hawkers, and are considered no better than vacuum salesmen, or worse. Because of this negative perception, female detail/drug reps are often subjected to inappropriate behavior on the job. The only time this author ever had an incident of sexual harassment in the workplace was as a pharmaceutical sales rep. One time, a hospital pharmacist called the author "no better than a prostitute." Other times, lewd remarks were made by the same physicians who had once treated the author in a respectful manner in other jobs *prior* to her employment in pharmaceutical sales.

Conclusion

In some ways, pharmaceutical companies are at odds with the American public. Many times, what's good for pharmaceutical companies is bad for consumers. In order to continue double- digit profits, keep stockholders and Wall Street happy, and employ tens of thousands of people, Big Pharma will have to extract maximum value from each product on the market. This is usually done by pricing at optimum levels, obtaining access to the market at an accelerated rate and maintaining unrestricted prescribing access. For consumers, our goals are completely the opposite: force the prices lower through appropriate legislation, encourage generic competition, create competition through Canadian pharmacies/Internet companies, push for deeper discounts for Medicare, Medicaid and Managed Care, fight to prevent abuse of patents and exclusivity arrangements, and restrict access on prescription drugs that have yet to be proven safe and effective in the long term. Big Pharma is being advised to fuse biotech, generics, and innovation. If they listen, we might have even *more* of a monopoly than we have already, which in turn will ultimately lead to higher prices.

It's not that pharmaceutical companies are the only corporations out there that are allegedly guilty of abuse. However, they are probably one of the most *transparent,* since consumers have paid so much of the prescription drug ticket. Consider that Americans can have hundreds of thousands of dollars in hospital bills with only a $250 deductible. Meanwhile, consumers continue to pay more out-of-pocket at their local drugstore. And although we *all* believe that pharmaceutical companies should concentrate their efforts on curing cancer and AIDS, the pharmaceutical company wouldn't keep making lifestyle drugs for baldness and impotence if consumers didn't want them and weren't willing to pay a high premium for them.

Perhaps Mark Merrill, president of the Pharmaceutical Care Management Association said it best: "the days of the drug industry dictating which drugs work, who should take them and what they should cost are *over.*"

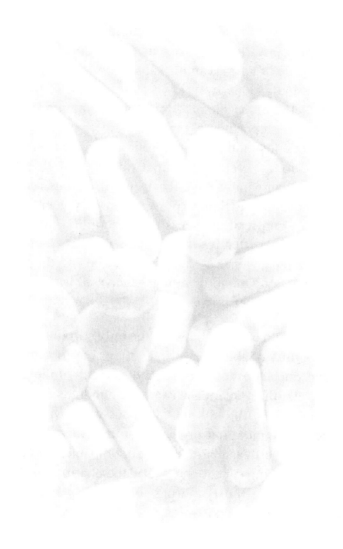

Chapter 6

HMOs and Insurance Prescription Drug Coverage- Your Rx to Relief

TIP: Get a copy of your healthcare plan's formulary and carry it with you to your doctor's appointments. Also, for chronic medications, use mail-order and save!

Introduction

Approximately 50% of Americans are fortunate enough to have prescription drug coverage through health insurance. Most Americans receive their health insurance from their employers, either through current employment or through employee retirement benefits.

This chapter was written to assist those readers who *have* prescription drug coverage through employer benefits. Even with a benefit, there are a maze of policies and procedures, benefit limitatio))ns and hoops to jump. (Note: the information in this chapter does not apply to individuals with drug coverage through Medicare, Medicaid, IHS, Federal Bureau of Prisons, Department of Defense, or Veterans Affairs.)

Many Americans don't realize what their health insurance coverage actually costs, since the employer pays the *majority* of the insurance premium, with only a small percentage paid by the employee. (The employee pays his/her portion of the premium through a pre-tax deduction.) According to the latest Kaiser Family Foundation survey, annual premiums for an HMO average $3,450 for a single employee or $9,504 for a famil)y plan. This is approximately a 6% increase. The employee's share of this amount is about 25-30% of the total.[1]

One of the reasons you see so much press about the cost of prescription drugs, is that prescription costs are rising at a disproportionate rate compared to other health care costs (approximately 10% for employees with family coverage.) HMOs and Insurance companies are asking consumers to shoulder a higher percentage of those costs through new reimbursement strategies. The days of the $5 copays for prescription drugs are over. According to IMS Health, copays averaged $5 for generics and $9 for non-preferred brands in 1996. By 2002, roughly 60% of healthcare plans, including HMOs, had raised the copays to an average of *$10* for generics and up to *$40* for non-preferred brands.[2] The average American still clings to the hope that most prescription drugs can be purchased with a very low copay. To quote Ken Sperling, a healthcare practice leader with Hewitt Associates: "They're on $10 copay island. They like it there and they don't want to leave."[3]

Not all employers provide health insurance. Federal laws require only companies with 20 employees or more to provide health insurance. Many employers cannot afford to offer health insurance and a majority of businesses have stated that it is their #1 business concern for 2005. For example, the large employer-General Electric- has reported spending more than $4.2 billion a year on health care costs, with $1.3 billion of the costs spent on prescription drugs. General Motors, who spends over 5 billion on health care states that for every new car, $1,225.00 of the vehicle's overall cost is needed to pay GM's employee health care benefits. *If* employers offer health insurance, prescription drug coverage is almost always part of the package. However, the extent of coverage, as well as the cost of the benefit, varies greatly from company to company. Large employers are urging workers to act more like shoppers. In other words, here is another large group who supports the purpose and concepts of this book.

Benefit designs/plans for HMOs and other managed care organizations (healthcare plans)

For purposes of this chapter and to allow for useful generalizations, all private insurance plans will be referred to as "healthcare plans." However, it might be beneficial to provide readers with basic definitions for the different *types* of healthcare plans. There is a saying in the health care industry: "If you've seen one HMO you've seen one HMO." There are many different insurance hybrids and benefit designs. Definitions and distinctions include:

1. HMO- (Health Maintenance Organization) - This is the most restrictive form of managed care organization in terms of health care services/accessibility and it is also the most affordable. An HMO provides health care to voluntarily enrolled members in return for a pre-set amount of money on a per member/per month basis. Members must use contracted providers in order for medical services to be covered.

2. PPO- (Preferred Provider Organization) - This is a very popular managed care plan that contracts with independent providers at a discount for services. These providers are known as "in-network" providers. Members have the option of seeing either in-network or out-of-network providers, but pay different out-of-pocket expenses for each.

3. POS- (Point-of-Service) - A POS is a managed care plan that contracts with a set of independent providers but allows members to use doctors and hospitals *outside* the plan for an additional cost. For example, POS providers would be reimbursed at 80-100% of charges but non-POS providers would be reimbursed at 70%.

4. IPAs- (Independent Practice Association)-This is an organization of physicians that has a contract with a managed care plan to deliver services in return for a pre-paid rate.

5. MCOs- (Managed Care Organization)- The term MCO was coined to describe all managed care plans such as HMOs, PPOs, POSs, etc.

6. Indemnity Insurance- This is the most expensive insurance because it allows members to go to any providers they choose and be reimbursed at the same levels. The traditional indemnity insurance requires the member to pay 20% of the charges, and the insurance company then pays 80%.

Drug benefit components

Components of drug benefit coverage that readers should understand include:

1. Copayments- This is the out-of-pocket portion of the prescription drug price that the employee/patient pays. Most of the time it's a set amount, not a percentage. For example, the $10-$40 a patient pays at the pharmacy is a copay. The actual cost of the drug is probably closer to $20-$90, but the employee is required to pay just a small portion of the total cost.

2. Co-insurance- This is the out-of-pocket portion of the price that the employee pays in a *percentage*, rather than a set dollar amount. (Usually it's 10-20% of the total price.) Depending on the prescription benefit, consumers can be responsible for a co-insurance payment alone or in combination with a copay, if the pharmacy is "out of network." An out-of-network pharmacy is a *non-participating* pharmacy for that specific employer or insur-ance; employees will usually pay more out-of-pocket when they use an out-of-network pharmacy.

3. "Tiered" programs- Tier means "levels or steps" for which pre-scription drug costs are reimbursed. Most tiered programs are 3-tier, meaning there are 3 different categories and each category has a different copay (or percentage). Tier 1 is usually the *Generic* drug category with the lowest copay-typically $10. Tier 2 is known as the *Preferred Brand* category, which includes brand name drugs that the healthcare plan believes are the best choices based on safety, efficacy, and cost. Tier 3 is the *Non-preferred Brand* category. These are the brand name drugs that are not believed to be the best choice in their therapeutic category (based on safety, efficacy and primarily cost) and they will therefore have the highest copay- as much as $40. Some plans have 4-tier programs, which includes a small number of brand name drugs at an even higher cost. Approximately 66% of drug benefit designs are now a 3-tier program, 23% are 2-tier, and only 13% have a

single or 1-tier copay.[4]

4. <u>Formularies</u>-A formulary is a drug list that is usually developed by the healthcare plan's own Pharmacy and Therapeutics (P & T) Committee. The P & T Committee consists of physicians, pharmacists and other healthcare personnel. Its purpose is evaluating the safety, efficacy, and overall value of prescription drugs, especially the new brand name drugs recently approved by the FDA. Some healthcare plans contract out for this service, but most have a P & T Committee in-house. There can be *closed* formularies where the healthcare plan doesn't pay for any prescription drug not on the list or *open* formularies where they might pay a portion of a drug not on their formulary.

5. <u>Mail-order</u>- Mail-order programs are used by plans as a cost savings strategy. Members typically order their drugs via fax, telephone, e-mail or the Internet. Ordinarily, only maintenance drugs for chronic conditions are available via mail-order and prescriptions are filled for a 90-day supply. (Note: not all prescription drugs will have a 90-day maximum supply; it depends on the drug). Employees gain the benefit of having to pay only 1-2 copays instead of 3. There is also the convenience of not having to make a trip to the pharmacy every month. Mail-order programs do a great job of filling prescriptions with generic substitutions. To participate in mail-order programs, employees will be required to complete an enrollment form (obtained by the healthcare plan) and a "Patient Profile." The main disadvantages to mail-order include waiting the 4-14 days for delivery from the time the order is mailed, and the hassle of getting a copy of the original prescription form directly from the physician to the mail-order pharmacy. However, most mail-order firms are more than willing to assist patients with obtaining prescription information directly from the physicians' offices. SOME EMPLOYERS, (INCLUDING GENERAL MOTORS & OTHER AUTO MAKERS), HAVE NOW INTRODUCED A MANDATORY MAIL-ORDER REQIREMENT FOR CHRONIC CONDITIONS.[5]

6. <u>Generics</u>- The use of generic prescription drugs is heavily encour-

aged. Besides saving the employee out-of-pocket costs, it also saves the employers in added health insurance costs. If fact, managed care organizations have been responsible for the continued increase in the volume of generic drugs sold. This is a very positive movement as generics are still the best value in both efficacy and price.

PBMs

Pharmacy Benefit Managers, or PBMs, are essentially intermediaries who administer prescription plans for employers and insurers. This is done to help control the rising prescription drug costs. PBMs have become especially significant in the last two decades; approximately two-thirds of all prescriptions written in the U.S. are processed by a PBMs.[6] There was a time when many of the major PBMs were actually owned by Big Pharma. This is like asking the rooster to watch the henhouse in that Big Pharm could then control both the supply and the demand of prescription drug purchases. In addition, a few PBMs were accused of accepting funds from drug manufacturers to switch customers' prescriptions from one drug to a completely different drug, without even obtaining the doctor's consent.

Thankfully, the PBMs that have survived are now independent and offer the following services and benefits:
1. Negotiates discounts and rebates for employers and insurers with the major pharmaceutical companies-Typically, PBMs retain a portion of the rebates in exchange for their services and then pass on the remainder of the savings to the healthcare plans/employers. However, once again, it allegedly instills a possible conflict of interest by steering physicians to prescribing drugs based *not* on efficacy but on discounts and rebates. (Discounts are usually based on volume.)
2. Offers mail-order pharmacies- PBMs can operate their own mail-order pharmacies or can contract out with separate companies. This is one service that passes on the savings to the consumers.
3. Conducts drug utilization review- this is the review of drug data

that looks for drug-drug interactions, drug allergies, contraindications and other red flags.

4. Provides formulary management- PBMs often assists the healthcare plans' P & T Committees in the review of new brand name drugs and provides valuable cost information.

5. Encourages use of generics- (generic substitution rates can be as high as 95% with the use of a PBMs.) PBMs can assist healthcare plans in implementing generic utilization programs, which in turn can cut drug costs dramatically.

6. Conducts disease management- Often referred to as case management, the programs are implemented by the PBMs in order to manage medical services (including prescription drug products) for patients with specific chronic diseases such as asthma, diabetes, and heart disease.

7. Creates "step therapy" programs- Step therapy is a set of guidelines that authorize specific drugs in steps-meaning that drugs that are less expensive are tried first and then if the disease is not controlled, different drugs in the next step can be authorized and covered. An example is step therapy for hypertension.

PBMs generally do not actually take possession of prescription drugs; they act as a go-between. However, in their mail-order and specialty-pharmacy businesses, PBMs do buy drugs from wholesalers or manufacturers and dispense them directly to patients in a manner similar to pharmacies.

As evidenced above, PBMs provide a valuable service and many believe their profits appear reasonable at around 3%. Names of the largest PBMs that employers are likely to use are:

- Medco Health Solutions
- Express Scripts
- Advance PCS/Caremark
- ACS State Healthcare

New strategies for controlling prescription drug costs

PBMs, managed care companies, and integrated delivery systems are creating new, innovative cost-cutting strategies. Consumers may like some of the strategies but dislike others. Examples include:

- Offering coupons (or vouchers) to waive the copayment for generic drugs: For example, Blue Cross/Blue Shield of Michigan provides coupons for generic versions of many commonly prescribed brands such as BuSpar for anxiety, Glucophage for diabetes, and Prinivil for high blood pressure. In a pilot of the program, BCBS of Michigan found that they saved $3 for every $1 spent on the program.

- Free Generics: The University of Wisconsin Hospital and Clinics developed a very innovative program; the program offers patient vouchers for free generics for a specified time in place of drug samples. Mr. Lee Vermeulen, Director of the Center for Drug Policy at the University of Wisconsin, estimates that for every $1,000 spent on generics, they will save *$1 million*-(note this cost savings is based on a full year of therapy with the generics rather than the branded alternatives.)[7]

- Excluding prescription drugs in a therapeutic class when an OTC is available: Historically, healthcare plans do *not* provide coverage for over-the-counter drugs, even when the cost might be considerably less than prescription drugs in the same therapeutic class. The idea is to shift the cost to the employee/enrollee, as soon as the drug is available over-the-counter (think Claritin and Prilosec). So, as strange as it seems to enrollees, one month prior to OTC-availability, a healthcare plan would cover the drug and the very next month it would be excluded; the decision has nothing to do with safety and efficacy, but rather with cost. This has been standard practice, but what *is* new is that some healthcare plans will no longer cover prescription drug alternatives *in the same therapeutic class as the OTC;* thereby forcing the patient to shoulder the cost, either with the prescription or the over-the-counter drug(s). An example of this strategy would be: a healthcare plan would not cover OTC Prilosec, nor would it cover Nexium or any other prescription drug in that therapeutic class.

An important note about copays

Since HMOs have continued increasing copayment amounts, many worry that it discourages patients from purchasing their prescriptions. A study co-funded by the Agency for Healthcare Research and Quality showed that "increasing copayments for prescription medications led to *decreases* in the use of 8 classes of therapeutic drugs." Based on this analysis, the researchers estimated that doubling copayments in a typical 2-tier drug plan resulted in an approximately 45% reduction in the use of anti-inflammatory drugs and antihistamines, a drop of approximately 35% in the use of cholesterol-lowering medications and drugs to treat ulcers and asthma····"[8] Some may believe that while the reduction in anti-inflammatory and antihistamine drugs may not cause severe health problems, reductions in treatment for cholesterol, and asthma carry great implications to personal and public health.

How to save money, even *with* prescription drug coverage

Even though a healthcare plan will pick up the majority of the costs of prescription drugs, there are some things that enrollees/patients can do to still be a savvy shopper:

1. Buy generic whenever possible. Remember to ask the health care practitioner (doctor, physician assistant, nurse practitioner) if he/she is writing for a generic version *when* he is writing the pre-scription. If it is not a generic, ask why not.
2. Ask the doctor if the prescription drug he is prescribing is on the healthcare plan's formulary- Physicians *should* know, or be able to verify, if the drug they are prescribing is on the formulary, but

sometimes they don't. Ultimately, it's up to the patient. Try to bring a copy of the formulary to all doctor's appointments. The healthcare plan should provide enrollees with copies of its formulary, either via mail or the Internet. In addition, if a patient is interested in asking a physician for a particular drug product (e.g. a drug seen in a TV Ad) the patient should check his/her formulary *prior* to the office visit in order to determine if it is even covered.

3. Call the pharmacy *prior* to dropping off the prescription to verify that it's in stock and that it is included in the Tier-1 copay category. If the pharmacist says no, ask why not. Make sure the reason is because there is no generic equivalent for the drug prescribed: that should be the only valid reason! (E.g. *not* because the pharmacy is out of stock or filling the prescription with a brand name drug out of habit, etc.)

4. If the prescription drug is not covered on the formulary, request a "prior authorization approval" from the health plan *prior* to purchasing. Many employees do not realize that if a drug the physician prescribes is not on their healthcare plan's formulary; they can still request approval through "prior authorization." However, the burden is placed on the *physician* to prove that the prescription drug is "medically necessary" and *not* on the patient. This can be a very time-consuming process but works best if the patient asks the physician to write a letter of "medical necessity" to the healthcare plan or insurance company. Whether the request is approved or denied, the employee and/or the physician should receive a letter from the healthcare plan on its decision. If the request has been denied, the last step is the appeals process…

5. Know the healthcare plan's APPEALS PROCESS-This is the employee's last recourse within the healthcare plan. Each healthcare plan has its own appeals process that is explained in its Member Handbook, as well as displayed on its website. The appeals process is inclusive of all covered medical services, including prescription drugs. There are many legal requirements that a health care plan *must* follow if the letter is an actual appeal. One requirement is that the healthcare plan must complete a time-

ly review. Many times the outcome is decided by a neutral party. If an employee has a legitimate case, *usually,* but not always, the decision will go in his or her favor. Studies show that 50% of the cases that are referred to neutral, outside panels are decided in favor of the patients.[9]

Here are the procedures the employee or the employee's representative should follow:

a. Call the healthcare plan and say "I am appealing my denied care."

b. Then put the appeal in writing. Make sure that the letter uses the word "appeal."

c. Send the letter by certified or registered mail, overnight delivery or fax, making sure to keep proof (e.g. receipts) that the correspondence was sent and preferably, received.

d. Follow the appeals process in the Member Handbook or website, if it differs from the above instructions.

6. Establish a relationship with a mass merchant, discount, or Internet pharmacy. If a patient winds up having to pay for the pre-

---

It Could Happen To You

A friend of the author's (Joan B) went to her local pharmacy to fill a prescription for the drug acyclovir, without checking first to see if it was on her healthcare plan's formulary- Turns out it wasn't, so Joan was charged the pharmacy's full price- $28.69 for 30 tabs for a generic! If Joan had referenced the formulary *first,* she would have known it was not covered under her insurance, at which time she could then have shopped around and called other pharmacies. For example, at Costco, the price was only $24.93 for 100 tabs! That's 25 cents a pill- vs. 96 cents a pill for 30 tabs at the chain pharmacy. Joan paid almost 4 times as much by not being prepared. Joan could also have chosen the prior-authorization process to obtain approval for the drug based on medical necessity and then could have paid just a $10 copay.

scription, the best price will be probably be through a mass merchant (e.g. Costco) or an Internet pharmacy such as www.drugstore.com. There are more drugs *not* on healthcare plan formularies than most people realize (see story below)

Conclusion

Americans who are fortunate enough to have prescription drug coverage are indeed the lucky ones. Those that do have prescription coverage should read their Member Handbook and obtain a copy of the healthcare plan's formulary as soon as possible. However, remember that not all drugs will be covered under their insurance. Preparing in advance for that actuality will save aggravation, as well as money.

Chapter 7

Drug Discount Cards (Non-Medicare)

> **TIP:** Since the discounts with cards are only 10-25% off retail, try Costco or www.drugstore.com instead. If using a discount card is preferred, call the card company first and get price checks on prescribed drugs prior to paying enrollment fees.

Introduction

This chapter has a different look and content from even just a year ago. This is because historically, drug discount cards were used primarily by seniors without prescription drug coverage. However, now that the Medicare Drug Discount Card Program is part of the new Medicare law and drug coverage is due to begin in January 2006; many of the standard drug discount cards are a non-issue. (Note: Drug Discount Cards for seniors with Medicare are covered in Chapter 8.)

For the 40 million uninsured Americans *without* prescription drug coverage, as well as all the Americans with l*imited* drug coverage, drug discount cards are still a viable option. In addition to the uninsured, some consumers use drug discount cards to supplement existing benefits (e.g. to pay for a prescription drug not on a healthcare plan formulary.) Drug card programs discussed in this chapter are **voluntary** discount programs, and may or may not be part of an insurance program (e.g. like the *AARP card*, which can be purchased with or without a Medigap policy.)

How it works: a consumer signs up for a "membership" with a specific Drug Discount Card Company and receives a special card to take to his/her local pharmacy. The discount is automatically applied to the purchase right *at the pharmacy*. It is a discount program, *not* an insurance program. However, it is similar to insurance in that not every pharmacy participates in every discount card program and cardholders must use a participating pharmacy to receive discounts.

What consumers *don't* realize is that the discounts are usually taken from the pharmacy's share of the sale, <u>not</u> from the drug manufacturer (e.g. Big Pharma). And on average, nearly 77% of the cost of the pharmaceutical dollar goes to the manufacturer, 23% to the pharmacy and the balance to the wholesaler/distributor. This is the reason that the discounts are rarely more than 10-20% of the total sale, which in turn may be why drug discount cards aren't more popular. However, it should be noted that the discounts might indeed be greater for some *generics*, based on contracts the pharmacy chains make with the manufacturers and/or distributors. Since most drug discount card programs require a $20-25 annual enrollment fee, there may be minimal savings if the number and type of prescriptions an individual purchases is limited.

Prescription drug discount card sponsors include, but are not limited to:
1. <u>Pharmaceutical companies</u>- some drug companies have created their own discount cards or have collaborated with several other companies to create a 'collective' card. They are very limiting, however, in that there are income restrictions, and frequently, age restrictions. In addition, the enrollee cannot have any other type of prescription drug benefit. And although their discounts may be comparable to other discount cards, their cards include *only* prescription drugs made by that specific pharmaceutical company(s). Due to the fact that most of the cards are for seniors only, (the Pfizer Pfriends Card is one exception), these cards will also be discussed in Chapter 8.
2. <u>PBMs</u>- many of the PBMs offer drug discount cards. The advantages to the PBM cards are that there are no age, insurance, or income restrictions (unless they are a Medicare discount card, an AARP card, or other.) They also cover most prescription drugs, not just the selected drugs made by one manufacturer.
3. <u>State Prescription Assistance Programs</u>-At least 25 states offer drug discount programs for seniors, low-income individuals and in some instances, state employees. (The state programs are discussed in Chapter 9.) Many of these programs have discount cards but they have age and/or income/eligibility requirements.

4. <u>Other for-profit companies</u>. Since virtually anyone can start a company that offers discounts on medical services, there are many other cards available that offer discounts on hospital admissions, physician visits, *and* prescription drugs. Due to the fact that the business is *not* an insurance product, the strict insurance rules and regulations do not apply. Some of these programs are legitimate; however, some are not. This is often another "buyer beware" scenario. Ads for these programs show up on TV and radio, as well as in junk e-mail.

Discount card savings

A study conducted by Brandeis University Schneider Institute for Health Policy in 2003 (*incidentally, funded by 4 PBMs*), showed: "actual discounts from prescription drug card programs administered by national PBMs for uninsured seniors are considerable, and vary depending upon generic or brand status and type of pharmacy. The average discount for generic medications was 26% and the average discount for brand drugs was 14%. The *overall* average discounted price for a prescription drug compared to the full retail price was 15%."[1]

Another study conducted by the General Accounting Office (GAO) showed varying amounts of discounts, but again, they were relatively small. In fact, a spokesperson at the GAO told Consumer Reports that consumers might save as much on their own if they work at it.[2]

Table 1: HOW MUCH MONEY CAN YOU SAVE?

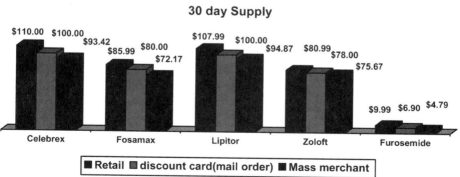

30 day Supply

Celebrex: $110.00, $100.00, $93.42
Fosamax: $85.99, $80.00, $72.17
Lipitor: $107.99, $100.00, $94.87
Zoloft: $80.99, $78.00, $75.67
Furosemide: $9.99, $6.90, $4.79

■ Retail ■ discount card(mail order) ■ Mass merchant

Note: This chart is for demonstration purposes. Prices vary and are subject to change.

Pros of discount cards
1. 10-25% discount off of full retail prices.
2. Purchases can be made at retail pharmacies and/or through mail-order pharmacies (usually the mail-order option is the better value.)
3. Valuable drug information is available through the cards' printed materials and on the companies' websites. Information includes product information, price checks, drug interactions, safeguards for drugs dispensed through the program, counseling from registered pharmacists and emergency access to pharmacists 24 hours a day.

Cons of discount cards
1. Not *all* pharmacies accept *all* discount cards.
2. EVERY PROGRAM HAS A FORMULARY, OR PREFERRED DRUG LIST. This means not *all* drugs will have discounts.
3. *Most* discount cards require a $20-$30 enrollment fee.
4. The discounts help, but again, are usually limited to 10-20% off full retail prices. For patients who can't afford an $80 drug purchase, a $60 prescription is probably not affordable either.

The best of the drug discount cards

The table on the following page displays a **comparison** of the best of the drug discount card programs, according to the author:

Name of Program	Benefits	Enrollment Fee	Contact & Misc. Info
YOURxPLAN- Medco	At 40,000 pharmacies	$25	www.yourplan.com or www. medcohealth.com 1-877-733-6765
AARP Member Choice (Note: This is the stand-alone program- Rx drug cards are free with enrollment into an AARP healthcare plan)	At 53,000 pharmacies, discounts on generics and brand name drugs-Average 17-47% and/or $189 annually	$19.95 if stand-alone	www.aarppharmacy.com 1-800-507-9622 Note: for AARP members (age 50+) only.
ScriptSave	At 95% of all pharmacy chains-Average 20% discount	None	www.scriptsave.com 1-800-347-5985 Anyone can join!

Conclusion

Drug discount cards can provide savings off of full retail prices and are therefore a viable option for consumers without prescription drug coverage. It is recommended that readers check with a couple of the card programs (i.e. those listed above) and ask about discounts for specific drugs *prior* to spending any money on enrollment fees. In addition, consumers should check to see whether their local pharmacies participate *prior* to enrolling. The author recommends ScriptSave, as it doesn't charge an enrollment fee, is open to everyone, and is an excellent program.

Keep in mind that there are probably better savings to be had through a mass merchant such as Costco or via a U.S. Internet pharmacy. However, using a discount card is still better than paying full retail price! See also APPENDIX A- Prescription Pathways- for more options.

For information on Medicare-approved Prescription Drug Discount Cards, please see the next chapter.

Chapter 8

Medicare & Senior Citizen Programs

> TIP: Check for Medicare Part D updates on the author's website:
> www.prescriptionpathways.com
> Check APPENDIX E in this book to get your user name and password.

Meet Mrs. Smith. Mrs. Smith is a 70-year-old female who lives in Phoenix Arizona. Her Social Security and Retirement Income is $1400/month. Her total assets, (excluding her home), are less than $10,000. She takes prescription drugs for osteoporosis, high cholesterol, gastroesophageal reflux disease, angina, and high blood pressure. She is currently taking Fosamax, fursoemide, Nexium, Lipitor and Norvasc. Her monthly prescription drug bill is $301.00 a month. Mrs. Smith's income is too <u>high</u> for her to qualify for public programs like Medicaid (called AHCCCS in Arizona), but too <u>low</u> for her to be able to afford a Medigap Policy.

Mrs. Smith is hoping that the government will soon pay for her prescription drugs. She knows it is not safe to buy drugs from Mexico and she is uneasy about buying drugs from Canada (via the internet) because she doesn't want to do anything illegal. Mrs. Smith wonders, what are her options?

Introduction

This chapter about Medicare has been entirely rewritten over the last 6 months, both literally and figuratively. Over the next two years, Medicare (and prescription drug coverage for seniors) is in the process of undergoing the single largest transformation in history. Thus, this chapter may be shorter and less comprehensive than many other chapters in this book. It focuses on what's happening *right now* as the book is published. Many more changes are ahead in 2005 and 2006 as the political wrangling over Medicare continues in Washington.

Since its inception in 1965, Medicare has been a huge slice of the U.S.'s health expenditures' "pie." Medicare provides insurance for more than 40 million elderly Americans. In 2001, Medicare expenditures totaled *$242 billion*. In other words, Medicare financed one-sixth of the U.S.'s overall health costs- and this was *without* the inclusion of a prescription drug benefit. Another government entitlement program, Medicaid, was almost that much with $224 billion in health care expenditures in 2001. (Medicaid is the federal/state program for low income and disabled individuals). While all medical expenditures for Medicare (and Medicaid) continue to increase, *prescription drug costs are rising at a disproportionate rate*. Rising prescription costs associated with Medicare recipients are also more publicized and *more politicized* due to the heavy burden that it has placed on the American public, especially for the portion of seniors with no prescription drug benefits.

Most Americans over 65, as well as many younger disabled individuals, have Medicare as their health insurance, but not *all* Medicare recipients have prescription drug coverage. As of 2004, approximately 15 million of America's seniors did *not* have any form of prescription drug coverage.

Some seniors have purchased supplemental insurance or have enrolled in Medicare managed care organizations (HMOs) in order to obtain prescription drug benefits. The following chart shows the breakdown of prescription drug benefits for Medicare recipients:

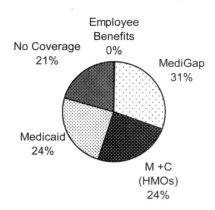

Prescription drug utilization for seniors

Consider the facts:

1. 90% of all older adults use at least 1 medication on a daily basis.
2. 40% use 5 or more medications daily.
3. 1/3 of prescriptions written in the U.S. are for the geriatric population.[1]
4. The average out-of-pocket prescription drug expenses for Medicare beneficiaries continue to rise. Seniors with prescription drug coverage pay approximately *$700/yr.* Those without coverage spend *$1,337/year* on average but out-of pocket spending quickly soars to $3,127 for those in fair or poor health. In addition, for the top 50 prescription drugs used most frequently by seniors, the *average annual* out-of-pocket cost as of January 2003 was $1,439.

The table below shows the <u>*average annual expenses*</u> for the last five years for <u>all</u> Medicare beneficiaries, *including those with and without* a prescription drug benefit.

Medicare Beneficiaries Out-of Pocket Prescription Drug Expenditures, 2000-2004

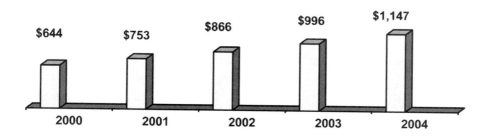

Medicare Prescription Drug Improvement Act and Modernization Act of 2003 (MMA)

A new beginning for Medicare and prescription drug benefits officially commenced on December 8, 2003, when President George W. Bush signed into law the _Medicare Prescription Drug Improvement and Modernization Act of 2003 (MMA)._ This new, massive 680-page piece of Medicare legislation added a prescription drug benefit, coverage for preventive services, and extra assistance for Medicare recipients with low incomes.

Even President Bush was quoted at a University lecture in Grand Rapids, Michigan as saying "Medicare and prescription drug coverage has long been used as a 'political football' by local and national politicians." And while many Americans were not completely satisfied with the final legislation that was passed (this author included), many still believe it is a step in the right direction. The question is this: is it better to have a flawed drug benefit rather than no benefit at all? That is the question on the minds of most seniors, as well as U.S. politicians, policymakers, advocacy groups and health care professionals.

To complicate matters even more, controversy swirled around the passing of the MMA, with accusations of possible bribes that Republicans allegedly offered to other house members to influence the vote on Medicare. For example, there were allegations that House Republicans offered one of the Republican congressional representative's money for his son's election campaign _if_ he voted for the Medicare legislation. (To date, nothing has been resolved regarding this accusation and others, and probably nothing will ever come of it.) There were also allegations that politicians misrepresented the actual cost of the MMA and that the price tag of $374 billion as presented to Congress and the public was wrong with the actual price tag closer to $700 billion! The financial estimates of the MMA keep rising every month. Over a 10-year period, the Medicare prescription drug benefit expenditures are expected to soar to almost $1 trillion! No one really knows; the only fairly accurate estimate is the $69.9 billion projected to be spent for Medicare Part D (prescription drugs) in 2006.

As of the publishing of this book, Medicare had increased its <u>premium</u> by 17.4% to $78.20/month in order to offset the additional benefits. This was the largest one-step increase since the program began in 1965. This is just the beginning of the changes that will be implemented as a result of the MMA. In addition, Medicare recipients' <u>annual deductibles</u> will increase in 2005 to $912 from $876. The higher out-of-pocket expenses may encourage consumers to look to switching to managed care/Medicare Advantage plans.

Medicare-approved Drug Discount Cards-The Stepping Stone!

As a stopgap measure prior to the implementation of the MMA (i.e. *actual* prescription drug coverage) in 2006, the legislation called for a Medicare-approved Drug Discount Card Program. The discount cards became effective in June 2004 and are to be used <u>until December 31, 2005.</u> Although the drug cards are considered a "benefit," it's really a discount program. The measure is truly just a stepping stone (some would just call it a "band-aid") until the true Medicare prescription drug benefit begins in 2006. Many have considered this program a failure since enrollment remained low throughout the first year of the program.

$600 credit for the Medicare-approved drug discount card program

One of the few true benefits of the Medicare-approved Drug Discount Card Program is the transitional assistance provided to low-income seniors and the disabled. Through the program, Medicare recipients who qualify were able to receive an annual credit of $600 for 2 years. (This is a maximum of $1,200 of free medications-although patients must still pay a 5%-10% coinsurance for every prescription.) Medicare recipients were eligible for the $600 credit if:
1. They had Medicare.
2. Their income was no more than $12,569 for a single person or no more than $16,862 for a married couple. (Note: income caps change every year because they are based on federal poverty levels.)

3. Different rules applied if they lived in Puerto Rico or a U.S. territory.
4. Medicare recipients must not have had Medicaid, TRICARE or any employer group health plan (e.g. employee retirement or union health coverage). Please note that if a Medicare recipient already had TRICARE or employee retirement benefits, then they probably already had prescription drug coverage and discussion of coordinating these benefits is beyond the purview of this chapter).
5. The credit would only be available through December 2005.

Generics and the card

Probably the greatest discounts realized with the drug discount cards have been with generics. A CMS study released June, 2004 that compared five generic drugs purchased with the discount card to the national average retail prices for the same generic drugs, showed discounts between 39% and 65% below the average prices paid at full retail. Although the majority of the top 50 drugs used by the elderly are brand name drugs, inexpensive generics are still a positive feature of the discount drug cards.

Small benefit to 50,000 people

Also in June 2004, the Bush administration announced that it would conduct a lottery to select 50,000 people to receive Medicare coverage until the MMA benefit became effective in 2006. These 50,000 Medicare beneficiaries would be receiving 28 expensive drugs used to treat cancer, rheumatoid arthritis, multiple sclerosis, hepatitis C and Paget's disease. It is estimated that there were approximately 500,000-600,000 people eligible to compete for the 50,000 slots (25,000 of them were cancer patients.[2]) Although this is a great benefit for cancer patients, it's not clear *what* the government thought this lottery system would accomplish since it was probably seen as systematic "rationing" of health care. Seniors who weren't fortunate enough to be picked for the lottery won't receive any assistance until 2006.

Card controversy

The Medicare-approved drug discount card program was very controversial from the outset. The rules were confusing; there were too many drug discount card options and seniors became victims of scams and frauds surrounding unapproved card programs. In 2004, a study conducted by the Kaiser Family Foundation, a non-profit health policy group, found that 53% of those surveyed agreed the cards weren't worth the trouble because the confusion was too high and the perceived benefit too low."[6] Seniors ranked the new drug discount card programs with an average "31" on a scale of zero to 100.[7]

By the time this book is published, the American public will have its "report card" on the drug cards and both the Federal government and the public will know exactly how effective this "band-aid" assistance really turned out to be. For the most part, the discount card program will soon be forgotten in order to make way for the real benefit in January 2006. (See information below.) For more information on the *drug discount card and the new benefit,* check the author's website at www.prescriptionpathway.com.

What to expect in 2006 when the MMA is a reality- prescription drugs will be covered!

As the MMA becomes effective in 2006, the following procedures will apply:

1. All Medicare recipients (referred to as "enrollees") will be able to enroll in plans that cover prescription drugs.
2. Enrollees will choose a prescription drug plan and pay a premium of about $37 a month.
3. Enrollees will pay the first $250 (called a deductible).
4. Medicare will then pay 75% of costs between $250 and $2,250 in drug spending. Enrollees will pay the remaining 25% of the drug costs.
5. Enrollees will pay 100% of the drug costs above $2,250 until they reach $3,600 in out-of-pocket spending. (This is what is known as the "donut hole.")

6. Medicare will then pay about 95% of the costs after enrollees have spent a total of $3,600. Enrollees will pay the remaining 5%.
7. Some prescription drug plans may have additional options to help enrollees pay out-of-pocket costs.
8. There will be extra help available for enrollees with *low incomes and limited assets.*
9. Starting in 2007, enrollees with incomes greater than $80,000 annually will pay higher premiums.
10. Medicare Advantage Plans (previously known as Medicare + Choice plans like those provided by PacifiCare, Cigna, and Aetna) will be expanded to include PPOs. PPOs will save enrollees money if they choose doctors and providers from a plan's "preferred list." Managed care companies will continue to offer HMO and Point-of-Service options as well. Healthcare plans will receive $46 billion in subsidies as an incentive to continue offering insurance products to seniors. (Incidentally, *Big Pharma* will probably benefit by $78 billion in additional revenues!)
11. Enrollees are not required to enroll in Medicare Advantage Plans in order to have a prescription drug benefit. Enrollees can choose to remain in the traditional Medicare plan and still receive prescription drugs (if they enroll in a prescription plan.)
12. The new benefit requires a formulary or list of preferred drugs. In other words, not all drugs will be covered. Medicare plans will be required to cover some, but not all, drugs in each therapeutic class. To date, there are approximately 140 different plans that will be offering the prescription benefit and conforming to formulary requirements. They will also be negotiating prescription drug prices.
13. **Four** Parts to Medicare!
    a. Medicare Part A- hospital care, skilled nursing facility care, home health care and hospice care.
    b. Medicare Part B- outpatient services such as physician visits, radiology, laboratory and outpatient hospital services. In addition, Medicare Part B also covers the following prescription drug categories: (approximately 32 drugs)

      i. Drugs that are not self-administered and furnished "incident" to a physician's service such as prostate cancer drugs;

     ii. Certain self-administered oral cancer and anti-nausea drugs;

   iii. Certain drugs used as part of durable medical equipment of infusion services (e.g. the Albuterol used in nebulizers, etc)

    iv. Immunosuppressive drugs, which are used following organ transplants

     v. Erythropoietin (EPO) to treat anemia and end stage renal disease and cancer patients;

    vi. Osteoporosis drugs furnished to certain beneficiaries by home health agencies.

> These drugs are typically provided in hospitals, dialysis centers, or doctor's offices and are purchased by the physician or hospital. In addition, Medicare Part B covers certain vaccines as well.

  c. Medicare Part C- Medicare Part C is the Medicare Risk Contract or HMO program, which has been called Part C or Medicare+Choice since 1997. It will be expanded and known as Medicare Advantage as of 2006.

  d. Medicare Part D- this is the new prescription drug benefit that has been added as a result of the Medicare Modernization Act.

Anyone confused yet?

Help for low-income seniors

The new Medicare drug benefit will provide additional assistance to low-income seniors. For individuals with Medicare and Medicaid coverage (known as "dual eligibles"), they will pay *no* premium or deductible, have *no* gap in coverage and pay just $1 per prescription for generics and $3 for brand name drugs. For people with incomes *between* 120-135%

of the poverty level ($12,919 for a single person or no more than $17,320 for a married couple) and assets *under* $7,500 for singles and $12,000 for couples, they will pay no premium or deductible, have no gap in coverage, and pay $2 for generics and $5 for brand name drugs. For people with incomes *below* 150% of the poverty level $14,355 and $19,245 and assets *under* $11,500 ($19,245 for couples), they will pay premiums on a sliding fee scale, a $50 deductible and 15% of drug costs with no gap in coverage.

Sound terribly confusing? It is… And these income levels will also change yearly. In addition, other policies could change in the next few years dependent on amendments that might be passed by Congress.

Any individuals who believe they might qualify for low-income subsidies should contact their State Health Insurance Assistance Program (SHIP). SHIPs are state programs that give free local health insurance counseling to people with Medicare. SHIP employees can also help answer questions regarding Medigap policies, long-term care insurance options, Medicare rights and appeals, claims, etc. For further information, call 1-800-Medicare and ask the customer representatives for the phone number of the appropriate state's SHIP.

Medicare Advantage Plans

Medicare Advantage (MA) Plans are the new managed care plans under MMA that will replace the existing Medicare+ Choice plans (e.g. Cigna, Aetna, and PacifiCare). In 2003, total enrollment in Medicare HMOs was down to 4.6 million nationwide from the high of 6.3 million in 1999. There were approximately 148 Medicare+Choice plans available in 2003, although more than 1 in 4 of the enrollees lived in California. Historically, a problem with Medicare HMOs has been that they have limited drug coverage.
1. Only 69% of the M+C enrolled Medicare recipients have drug coverage.
2. Of those that offer drug coverage, 60% cover only generics.
3. More than 4 in 10 enrollees had an annual benefit prescription cap of $750 or less.[4]

Due to the new MMA law, it's unclear what the benefits will actually be for MA enrollees; however, physician choices will be expanded since there will be PPOs and POSs in addition to HMOs. Prescription drug coverage will also be expanded to cover the same (or better) benefit as the one offered to seniors in the traditional Medicare plan. The government expects managed care membership to triple to approximately 14.7 million people in the next three years which encompasses more than one in three elderly people.[5]

All Medicare recipients enrolled in Medicare Advantage Plans will be eligible for a prescription drug benefit. The MA plans may also choose to continue to offer additional services such as vision benefits, as they have done previously. In addition, they may continue refunding a portion of the monthly Medicare premium.

Is the Medicare MMA drug benefit worth it?

There has been a swill of controversy surrounding the true financial benefits as well as the costs of the MMA, especially regarding the prescription drug coverage. Many found fault with the construction of the law and found it "too friendly" to Big Pharma for several reasons, primarily because of the donut hole and the lack of provisions for the federal government to negotiate discounts or rebates from the pharmaceutical companies. Some believe savings of up to 1/3 of a billion dollars or more could have been realized by implementing discounted reimbursement formulas.

One excellent source for *each* individual to determine the *value* of the drug benefit is the AARP website: www.aarp.com. From the website, click on "Medicare Rx Information" and then click on "Benefit Calculator." Then type in the total dollar amount spent annually on prescription drugs, and click "Calculate." This will enable Medicare recipients to determine what the actual cost savings will be. For instance, if a Medicare patient spent $400 annually on prescription drugs prior to the drug benefit, the new out-of-pocket costs would actually be *more*: $707.50. This is due to the cost of the annual premium, deductible, co-insurance, etc. However, if a patient spent $1400 annually, that patient would only spend $957.50

per year with the new benefit and thus save $442.50 annually.
The website: www.medicare.gov

The best source for all the specific policies of the new Medicare law is the Federal government's website: www.medicare.gov. Here Medicare recipients will find information on drug discount cards as well as the new Medicare prescription drug benefit. The website also includes a drug price comparison tool that not only lets individuals see current prices of existing prescription drugs, but also gives them several lower cost options of drugs in the same therapeutic *class*. (Note: the drugs used in the comparison may <u>not</u> be therapeutically equivalent (i.e. identical). Please be advised that medical advice concerning switching from one prescription drug to another should only be provided by a patient's individual physician.

Purchasing prescription drugs from Canada

Buying prescription drugs from Canada has continued to remain a common practice among seniors *with or without* a prescription drug benefit. Again, this is because <u>no</u> single policy or program fully funds *100%* of all prescriptions. This is not going to change with the new Medicare benefit, either. Since Medicare is implementing a formulary, (a list of approved drugs), <u>there will be prescription drugs that seniors still have to purchase at full price</u>. In addition, there are gaps in coverage. Seniors will probably continue to purchase prescription drugs in Canada in these instances. (For more information on purchasing prescription drugs from Canada, refer to Chapter 13.) The problem with purchasing prescription drugs from Canada for the "donut hole" is that Medicare recipients cannot count these expenditures towards their annual purchases in order to be "bumped up" into the catastrophic category. They then remain in the "black hole" of the "donut hole" until the following calendar year, when the process starts all over again!

For readers who are *not* enrolled in Medicare

If an individual is a senior but is *ineligible* for Medicare, he or she should contact the local State Assistance Program (SHIP) and ask for locations of "safety net" providers and community health centers in the area. Community health centers are wonderful health care centers that can provide medical services and prescription drugs at sliding fee scales and discount prices for uninsured seniors and the disabled.

Another source of assistance is the website www.benfitscheckup.com. This website is sponsored by the American Council on Aging. This website asks approximately 35 questions to help an individual determine what, if any, prescription drug coverage and health insurance is available in to them based on income, age, gender, etc. If a senior is ineligible for Medicare, this can be a useful website.

In addition, if an individual is over 64 ½ and will be turning 65 within the next six months, this individual should contact the Social Security Administration at (800) 772-1213 to avoid any lapses in health care coverage and to avoid Medicare's penalty for late registration. Medicare enrollment usually does not occur automatically. In addition, there are strict enrollment periods and enrollment procedures for Medicare Part B and Medigap Policies. For additional information, see the website www.medicare.gov or call 1-800-Medicare.

Specific prescription drugs seniors should not use

Due to chronic diseases and certain conditions related to aging, seniors have additional problems with taking some prescription drugs. Problems arise from adverse drug reactions and inappropriate prescribing. Adverse drug reactions occur in 10-35% of older adults, due to many factors relating to absorption, distribution, metabolism, and excretion.[6] This happens more often than it should. According to findings reported in the Journal of the American Association, about 1/5 of the approximately 32 million elderly Americans not living in nursing homes in 1996 used a least 1 of the 33 prescription medicines considered potentially inappropriate.[7]

Recently, the U.S. General Accounting Office (GAO) compiled a list of 20 drugs generally "considered inappropriate" for the geriatric population. Seventeen of the 20 drugs have been associated with medication errors submitted to MEDMARX^{SM} (see Chapter 3). Seniors need to be aware of this list; *however, inclusion on the list does <u>not</u> automatically preclude a patient's personal physician from prescribing them when the benefits of the drugs outweigh the risks.*

Any patient currently taking one of these medications should talk to his or her physician prior to discontinuing any drug therapy. The list includes:[8]

Diazepam
Amitriptyline
Chlordiazepoxide
Trimethobenzamide
Indomethacin
Dipyridamole
Proxpoxyphene
Cyclobenzaprine HCL
Methocarbanol
Phenobarbital
Carisoprodol
Flurazepam
Orphenadrine
Pentazocine
Chlorpropamide
Meprobamate
Cyclandelate

Consumer Information

The most valuable source for all things Medicare is the website: www.medicare.gov. Readers can also call 1-800-MEDICARE (1-800-633-4227).

Another great source for Medicare information is a handbook printed by U.S. Department of Health and Human Services that explains the

Medicare program, including the prescription drug benefit. It's entitled: "Medicare & You." This handbook is available in a paper book or on audiotape in both English and Spanish. Medicare will automatically be mailing the handbook to all recipients prior to January 2006. In the meantime, to receive a copy, call 1-800-MEDICARE and ask for the National

---

It Could Happen To You

Readers may remember Mrs. Smith who is discussed at the beginning of the chapter. So what would the drugs have cost her if she had signed up for the new Medicare Prescription Drug Discount Card? Well, she probably would not have been eligible for a discount. However, here is the good news. For the *new* Medicare Part D benefit beginning in January 2006, she will actually qualify for low-income subsidies because her income is less than $14,355 and her assets are under $11,500! Mrs. Smith is one of the 7 million seniors/disabled that this benefit will actually help. The best news for those that qualify- NO DOUGHNUT HOLE!

Medicare Handbook, "Medicare & You."

Conclusion

BOTTOM LINE: THERE IS NO PRESCRIPTION DRUG BENEFIT AVAILABLE ANYWHERE THAT WILL COVER 100% OF ALL PRE-SCRIPTION DRUGS AND 100% OF THE COSTS. Although many seniors believe that the new Medicare coverage would be all-inclusive, it won't. It may never be. This is all the more reason that seniors, with the assistance of their family, health care providers and pharmacists, must learn how to comparison-shop for the best prescription drug prices.

There is the adage that some help is better than no help, but many debate that wisdom because they see the MMA as a political ruse to turn the Medicare program into a senior entitlement program for the elderly poor. There are many areas of concern, especially relating to the Medicare disabled. But probably the most worrisome aspect of the new MMA is what will happen to seniors who now have employer-sponsored benefits. Many worry that the law will be a way out for Corporate America who no longer wants to offer health care benefits for retirees. Currently, employer-sponsored health care is the leading source of prescription drug coverage for seniors (28% of all Medicare recipients have prescription drug coverage through employer-sponsored benefits.[9]) Under the MMA, 86 billion in tax money will be given to employers as incentives if they continue offering benefits; however there are no guarantees that they will.

This book was designed to provide assistance when the federal and private governments leave consumers, including seniors, with gaps and out-of-pocket drug expenses. APPENDIX A provides a cost comparison for use in comparison-shopping. Readers can also go to the author's website: www.prescriptionpathway.com for all the newest updates on the MMA (including low-income subsidies) as well as for cost savings tips.

Chapter 9

Pharmaceutical Assistant Programs (PAPs)

> TIP: Go to the website: www.rxassit.org to determine if you qualify for free prescription drugs (based on your income). Rule of thumb is that standard income limits are approximately 16-18k/yr for singles and 25k/yr for couples.

Introduction

Currently in the U.S., it's a sad state of affairs for low-income Americans: those who are among the poorest *actually pay the highest cost for prescription drugs*. This is because many Americans who might otherwise qualify for government or private assistance purchase prescription drugs at local pharmacies *at the highest retail prices*. Studies have shown that *uninsured* consumers pay, on average, 72% more than other groups for the 10 most common prescription drugs.[1]

In the past few years, *hospitals and physicians* have stepped up to the plate to grant deep discounts on medical services to uninsured patients. Pharmaceutical companies on the other hand, have offered their solution for low-income and uninsured individuals with what they call "**Patient Assistance Programs**" or "**PAPs**." The pharmaceutical companies enjoy bragging that they provide drug products to over 6.2 million patients for 17 million prescriptions totaling over $1.5 billion/year. The 17 million prescriptions, however, amounts to less than 1% of the 3.5 billion prescriptions filled in 2003 and less than 1% of the total $217 billion revenues per annum.

At present, PAPs are the only option for *free* prescription drugs for individual Americans, unless they are fortunate enough to receive drug samples or are provided limited supplies of medications at free clinics or community health centers.

How Patient Assistance Programs work

First of all, it's important to know from the outset that Patient Assistant Programs (PAPs) are set up to be the "option of last resort." This means that if a consumer can qualify for Medicaid or any other public assistance, and just hasn't gotten around to it, or doesn't know how to sign up, or has been disenrolled but is eligible to re-enroll, then he/she will not be eligible for PAP assistance. In addition, if a consumer is an undocumented immigrant, has partial prescription drug coverage, but has reached his/her dollar limit or a particular drug(s) is not on the managed care formulary, PAPs are not an option. PAP programs are really geared towards a financial "notch" group that earns *too* much to qualify for Medicaid, but whose income is low enough that they can't afford to buy prescription drugs and/or healthcare insurance. It is not a panacea, a free ride or even easy. Many are of the opinion that Big Pharma makes it intentionally extremely difficult to participate in PAP programs.

General income guidelines for PAPs are roughly $18,000 year for single individuals and $25,000/year for couples. The income guidelines are based roughly on the equivalent of 150-200% of the poverty level. There are approximately 29 million Americans that could benefit from prescription PAPs. However, *exact* income requirements vary from program to program. In addition, they continue to change every year as the poverty level is adjusted. Approximately 1/3 of all the programs require some type of financial documentation, which may be a tax return, W2 and/or a payroll/check stub.

PAPs require massive time and paperwork and all of the programs have different application forms, different eligibility requirements and different procedures. There are over *160* PAPs operated by 80+ pharmaceutical companies, with over *800* medications included. The first time a patient is approved, he or she usually receives a 1-3 month supply. When it's time for a refill, the pharmaceutical companies will either renew the prescription automatically, or require that the patient start the application process over again.

Most of the drug companies have a requirement that medications must be sent to the physician's office and not to the patient's home; however, some will ship to a patient's home or provide vouchers instead (see details later in this chapter).

If an individual has *Medicare*, the pharmaceutical companies will first direct the individual to the Medicare Prescription Drug Discount Card Program. Presumably, when the Medicare Prescription Benefit is implemented in January 2006, Medicare patients will no longer be eligible for PAP assistance. For more information, Medicare recipients can also check the Medicare website (www.medicare.gov) and click on "Prescription Drug Assistance Programs" to view available pharmaceutical company-sponsored prescription assistance programs. At this website, there are three ways to obtain additional information on PAPs: 1) select up to 5 pharmaceutical company names to view available programs and/or 2) select up to five health conditions or diseases or 3) click "View Default Results." Readers can also check the website: www.pparx.org.

The application process

The application process for PAPs can be very difficult, time-consuming, and confusing. The application process requires the following steps:

    1) Check first to determine if the prescription drugs prescribed are included in one of the 160+ programs. *Use one of the three websites listed below.*

    2) Locate & complete application form- if allowed, the *patient* should complete the form. If the *physician* is required to complete the form, the patient should take a *blank* copy of the form and the corresponding mailing/fax/phone instructions to his or her physician's office for completion.

    3) Obtain a written prescription from the physician for a 3-month or 6-month supply.

    4) Mail or fax the following documents: application form, prescription form, and proof of income, if required (i.e. some companies require tax forms, a W2, or other forms of income verification).

5) Check back with the physician's office after a few weeks to determine if the medications have arrived. If the application is denied, the pharmaceutical company won't necessarily provide notification.

Do it yourself

If patients have access to the Internet, they can go online to complete the above Steps 1 & 2 themselves. Although each one of the three websites below have a phone number as well, it is much easier to complete the process via the Internet. The following three websites are recommended:

1) www.assist.org: This is a website created by Volunteers in Health Care, a national program supported by the Robert Wood Foundation. It comes equipped with a database that allows both patients and physicians to search for PAPs by company, brand name, generic name, and drug class. The information presented also includes eligibility and application instructions and forms to download. The reason this website is rated #1 by the author is because it's not owned or managed by any pharmaceutical organizations and it assists patients with receiving both brand name _and_ generic drugs. It includes a new, very innovate program available called _Rx Outreach._ ™ This is a program that provides approximately 50 popular generic drugs to low-income and uninsured individuals. Unlike most of the brand name programs, the medications are mailed directly to patients. The cost of any of the generics is $18 for a 3-month supply and $30 for a 3-month supply. That amounts to only $5-$6 a month!

2) www.pparx.org- Partnership for Prescription Assistance- (also available at the website: www.helpingpatients.org). This is a program/website created by the pharmaceutical industry and serves as a centralized database for all of the programs. It includes the 80+ pharmaceutical company programs, as well as other public and private programs such as Medicaid, and Medicare. The information is categorized by state, but not every state is participating at the present time. To use the website, log on. Click "Patients" and then type in the brand name

of the prescribed drug(s). To review all programs in a particular state, go to: "Find your State."

3) www.rxhope.org: This is a good website for patients who want to conduct a quick 'Search' to see if their specific prescription medications are covered under a PAP. It will give the address and phone number of the pharmaceutical company so that patients may call them directly and ask them to walk them through the eligibility and enrollment process.

Aid from non-profit organizations

Any physician can complete PAP applications on a patient's behalf, however many private physician offices choose not to participate due to the labor-intensive nature of the process. Statistics show that physician offices can spend up to *11 hours per week* on PAPs, without any reimbursement from government agencies, insurance companies or the pharmaceutical industry. Sometimes, if a patient has done all the legwork and just asks the physician to complete and fax the form, they will comply.

On the other hand, community health centers and clinics that focus on providing care to the uninsured will almost always assist patients in enrolling in PAPs; Community Health Centers and Clinics provide medical services such as medical, dental, behavioral health and pharmacy as well as case management services. For community health center/clinic locations, log on to the National Association of Community Health Centers' website at www.nachc.com.

If an individual does not have Internet access, or finds the application process too confusing, a PAP service is available for a small fee. For a $5 per prescription fee, the Medicine Program, a non-profit organization, will do the research and forward all the documents (with instructions) directly to the individual. They can be contacted at (573) 996-7300 or at www.themedicineprogram.com,

Big Pharma with PAPs

As of July 2004, there were <u>11</u> PAPs sponsored by pharmaceutical companies that provided *vouchers* or cards for patients to redeem directly at the local pharmacies. Vouchers or cards are the **preferred** method due to ease of use. Companies with voucher/card programs include:

AAI Pharma, Inc.
Axcan Scandipahrm, Inc.
Bayer Pharmaceuticals, Inc.
Cephalon, Inc.
Chiron Corporation
Eisai, Inc.
GlaxoSmithKline
Janssen Pharmaceuticals
Nation Organization for Rare Disorders (NORD)
Novartis Pharmaceuticals

Other major pharmaceutical companies that have PAPs are listed below. (Note: this is only a *partial* list consisting of some of the larger companies.) Over 129 of the programs insist that the medications be sent directly to the physician office or advocacy center; only 29 of them allow the medications to be shipped directly to the patients' homes:

Abbott Laboratories
Amgen Inc.
AstraZeneca
Aventis Pharmaceuticals
Bristol-Myers Squibb
Genentech, Inc.
Merck & Co., Inc.
Pfizer Inc.
Schering-Plough
Searle
Eli Lilly and Company

State PAPs

Over the past decade, many states have created **State** Pharmaceutical Assistance Programs. The programs were primarily developed for seniors without prescription drug coverage, but some programs also include the disabled and the uninsured. As of July 2004, 39 states had established or authorized some type of program. At that time, 31 were operational and 31 offered a direct subsidy utilizing state funds. Other states have created programs that offer a discount only (no subsidy) for eligible seniors. All the state programs vary widely in eligibility (both financial and age related), coverage and operations.

Some of the states are now providing programs for purchasing prescription drugs from Canada for seniors, uninsured, disabled, and government employees.

For more information on State PAPs, there are many good websites and other references. Readers can contact their State Health Insurance Program, or visit the Medicare website at www.medicare.gov. Other good websites include: www.pparx.org as listed above, as well as www.ncsl.org/programs/health/drugaid.htm and click on "Public User".

Conclusion

In conclusion, PAPs are a viable option for low-income U.S. citizens that meet the very narrow eligibility requirements. For this group of individuals, it's probably one of our health care system's *best-kept secrets*! However, as a reminder, to receive benefits from any PAP, individuals must first exhaust every other avenue (e.g. Medicare, Medicaid, other state programs).

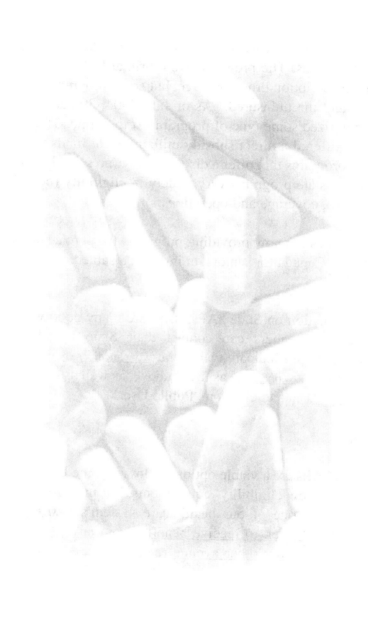

Chapter 10

Over-the-Counter (OTC) Medications

> **TIP:** Ask your pharmacist about any OTC product you buy; the pharmacist can tell you if the product is right for you. If you buy the OTCs often, comparison shop, use coupons and/or buy at a mass merchandiser store.

Introduction

Over the Counter (OTC) medications are defined as non-prescription medicines that have been proven safe enough by the FDA to be used without a physician's prescription order. Anyone can purchase OTC medications at local drugstores, grocery stores, warehouse stores, convenience stores, and gas stations and even on the Internet. Global sales of OTC products in 2002 were estimated to be *$47 billion!*

There are more than 100,000 OTC drugs commercially available. They contain approximately 700 active ingredients in more than 54 categories. Americans buy **5 billion** OTC products each year! This is 60% of all the drugs sold in the U.S. (i.e., *more OTC drugs are sold than prescription drugs*). In fact, 40% of the U.S. population consumes at least *one* OTC drug within any given 48-hour period and 73% of consumers prefer to treat symptoms themselves with OTC medications rather than with prescription drugs.[1]

OTC medicines treat an expanding range of ailments such as aches, pains, itches, allergies, etc. Overall, OTCs can be used to treat over 450 medical conditions.[2] Of the 3.5 billion health problems treated annually, 2.0 billion (57%) are treated with one or more OTC medications as primary or major adjunctive therapy.[3] Some can even *prevent* diseases such as tooth decay and athlete's foot, and many others *manage* diseases such as migraines, minor pain in arthritis, heartburn and rhinitis. Many of the

OTC medications treat the *same* conditions that stronger prescription drug alternatives treat, but without the need of a prescription (i.e. arthritis can be treated with Advil or Motrin but can also be treated with expensive prescription drugs such as Vioxx or Celebrex).

There are generic brands of OTCs just as there are generic brands of prescription drugs. For example, the Kroger brand found at Fry's is the store (generic brand) for many drugs such as the brand name drugs: Aspirin, Motrin, Claritin, etc. Just as with prescription drugs, OTC drugs made by generic manufacturers are regulated and monitored by the FDA and are equally effective but usually less expensive, *unless* the brand version is on sale.

OTC medicines are especially significant for the elderly since OTCs treat many of the aches, pains, and illnesses most likely to appear in our later years. Adults age 65 and older consume *1/3* of the OTC products in the U.S. Four out of five older Americans report at least one chronic condition and many of those conditions are treated with an OTC medication. According to the FDA and the Consumer Healthcare Products Association, "As we live longer, work longer, and take a more active role in our own health care, the need grows to become better informed about self-care."

Medicines that don't require a prescription have been around for centuries. For example, ASPIRIN (acetylsalicylic acid, a chemical originally used in dyes) is an OTC drug and truly a miracle drug; it can be purchased for just pennies a day. Bayer, the first company to make aspirin, introduced the product in 1900! Aspirin was originally manufactured to treat headaches and other aches and pains and is still used for those symptoms today. However, with further study, Aspirin has been found to improve heart health and is now taken by *$26 million* Americans every day to help prevent heart disease.

The top 10 OTC medicines by sales in 2001 were:
1. Private label internal analgesic tablets
2. Tylenol internal analgesic tablets
3. Private label cold/allergy/sinus tablets/packets
4. Advil internal analgesic tablets
5. Nicorette anti-smoking gum
6. Aleve internal analgesic tablets
7. Private label first-aid ointments/antiseptics
8. Benadryl cold/allergy/sinus tablets/packets
9. Nicoderm CQ anti-smoking patch
10. Private label antacid tablets.

It's virtually impossible to write a book about prescription drugs without also discussing OTC drugs, because *today's* prescription drugs are *tomorrow's* OTC drugs. Some of the top-selling drugs of the past few years like Claritin and Prilosec are now available over-the-counter and many more are expected in the next decade. The line continues to blur between prescription drugs, brand and generic, non-prescription drugs and dietary supplements. Consumers need to be informed about all these type of medications, especially when they are taken together.

Are OTC's Safe?

The FDA estimated in 2002 that more than __700__ OTC products on the market today use ingredients and dosages that were available only by prescription 20 years ago.

The FDA must determine that a prescription drug is "safe" before it can be switched from a prescription drug to an OTC. "Safe" means that the FDA has determined that a drug is safe enough to be sold directly to consumers over the counter. Sometimes when a prescription drug becomes an OTC, the lower doses of the drug are switched to OTC, but the higher doses still require a prescription.

It is important to remember that OTC drugs required a prescription and physician monitoring *not too long ago;* therefore OTC medications should be treated with the proper amount of respect in regards to safety.

Tampering

Due to the fact that OTC medicines are found right on the retail shelf, they are easily accessible and vulnerable to tampering. Six tips to protect against OTC tampering are:

1. Read the label and be alert to the tamper-evident features on the package *before* you open it.
2. Inspect the outer packaging for signs of tampering *before* you buy a product.
3. Examine the medicine before taking it. Checks for capsules or tablets that differ from the others. Do not use medicine from packages with tears, cuts, or other imperfections.
4. Never take medicine in the dark.
5. Examine the label and the medicine every time you take it or give it to someone.
6. Tell somebody (pharmacist or store manager) if a product doesn't look right.

According to a survey commissioned by the National Council on Patient Information and Education (NCPIE), some Americans do <u>not</u> take OTC medications correctly. This can lead to serious problems and is probably the main reason for drug side effects and drug interactions. The 2003 survey found:

- 51% of the respondents indicated they had taken an OTC and a prescription drug simultaneously
- 48% of the respondents had taken more than the recommended dose and;
- 35% of the respondents had taken the next dose of an OTC sooner than directed on the label.[4]

It is thought that probably one reason consumers don't take OTCs correctly is that there is a lack of understanding about how potent and potentially dangerous OTCs can be without proper supervision and safety measures.

The U.S. Surgeon General Richard Carmona, MD, MPH, and the National Council on Patient Information and Education (NCPIE) have produced a simple yet important educational tool for consumers regarding OTC medicines. It is listed below in its entirety:

MedWise Prescription for Taking Over-The-Counter Medicines with Care

When selecting an over-the-counter (non-prescription) medicine, always read the instructions and warnings on the product label. If you want more information, talk to your pharmacist or doctor.

Some Questions to ask:

- WHAT over-the-counter (OTC) medicines are available for the symptoms I want to treat?
- HOW much of this OTC medicine should I take at a time?
- HOW often should I take this OTC medicine?
- HOW many days in a row should I use this medicine to treat my symptoms
- WHAT other medicines (OTC and prescription), herbal products, or dietary supplements should I avoid while taking this OTC medicine?"

Remember, OTC drugs are serious medicines that should be taken with care, understanding the potential dangers if taken incorrectly or without counseling and education.

153

Drug Facts

The drug information found on the packaging of any OTC drug is also regulated by the FDA and is known as the "Drug Facts." *Drug Facts labels contain proper use information and should always be reviewed thoroughly.* Drug Facts must contain:

- Active Ingredient (for each tablet, dose)- chemical compound
- Uses- symptoms the medicine is approved to treat
- Warnings-what other medications, foods or other conditions to avoid while taking the OTC drugs (e.g. avoid driving)
- Directions – daily dose what and how often to take it. Follow these instructions to the letter.

A copy of the Drug Facts Label found on OTC antihistamine is illustrated below:

Drug Facts

Active ingredient (in each tablet)   **Purpose**
Chlorpheniramine maleate 2 mg ....Antihistamine

Uses temporarily relieves these symptoms due to hay fever or other upper respiratory allergies:
■ sneezing   ■ runny nose   ■ itchy, watery eyes   ■ itchy throat

Warnings
Ask a doctor before use if you have
■ glaucoma ■ a breathing problem such as emphysema or chronic bronchitis
■ trouble urinating due to an enlarged prostate gland

Ask a doctor or pharmacist before use if you are taking tranquilizers or sedatives

When using this product
■ you may get drowsy   ■ avoid alcoholic drinks
■ alcohol, sedatives, and tranquilizers may increase drowsiness
■ be careful when driving a motor vehicle or operating machinery
■ excitability may occur, especially in children

If pregnant or breast-feeding, ask a health professional before use.
Keep out of reach of children. In case of overdose, get medical help or contact a Poison Control Center right away.

Directions

adults and children 12 years and over	take 2 tablets every 4 to 6 hours; not more than 12 tablets in 24 hours
children 6 years to under 12 years	take 1 tablet every 4 to 6 hours; not more than 6 tablets in 24 hours
children under 6 years	ask a doctor

Other information store at 20-25° C (68-77° F) ■ protect from excessive moisture

Inactive ingredients D&C yellow no. 10, lactose, magnesium stearate, microcrystalline cellulose, pregelatinized starch

> ### Note
>
> If you're taking more than one OTC medicine, compare the active ingredients. Do not take two medicines with the same active ingredient unless instructed by your doctor, pharmacist or other healthcare professional.

Source: National Council on Patient Information's website: www.bemedwise.com

Other important safety reminders

Other important safety reminders can be found in the FDA /CPHA brochure entitled "Over-the-Counter Medicines- What's Right for you"? They are as follows:

Children

Approximately 1/3 of all OTC medicines purchases are for children. Additional precautions should be taken when giving children OTC medicines, including the following:

1. Follow age limits on the label (don't just estimate the dose based on size).
2. Know the difference between TBSP (tablespoon) and TSP (teaspoon) and use measuring spoons and not common kitchen spoons.
3. Before you give your child two or more medicines at a time, talk to your doctor or pharmacist.
4. Never call medicine candy to get your kids to take it. If they come across the medicine on their own, they're likely to remember that you called it candy and may take it without permission.
5. Child Resistant Packaging helps protect your children, but only if you *lock and close the bottles correctly*. However, the law allows one package size for each OTC to be sold without child-resistant features and this is acceptable if you don't have children and you find the child resistant packing difficult to use.

Pregnancy and Breast Feeding

Drugs can pass from a pregnant woman to her unborn baby and a safe amount of medicine for the mother may be too much for the unborn baby. If you are pregnant, always talk with your doctor before taking any drugs, prescription, and OTC and/or dietary and herbal supplements.
In regards to breast-feeding, most drugs pass through breast milk in low enough concentrations to not have any unwanted effects on the baby who is being breast-fed. However, always check with your doctor or pharmacist before taking any OTCs while breast-feeding.

Medicine Cabinet Checkup

Medication cabinets should be checked every 6-12 months. Discard any OTC medications that have expired or are no longer needed. OTC medicines, like *all* medications, lose their potency (effectiveness) over time. Take all expired products to a hazardous waste disposal facility. Also, OTC meds should be kept in their original container in the medicine cabinet, and out of the reach of any children.

Drug Interactions

The possibilities of drug interactions need to be taken into consideration when taking OTCs, especially when used in conjunction with prescription drugs. The American Pharmacists Association has developed a great brochure regarding drug interactions: "What You Should Know About Over-the-Counter Medicines and Drug Interactions." Information includes:
The three main kinds of drug interactions:
1. Drug-drug interactions- this occurs when two drugs interact. For example both aspirin and blood thinners like warfarin (Coumadin) help to prevent blood clots from forming. Using these medications together may cause excessive bleeding.
2. Drug-food interactions: This happens when a prescription or OTC medications interacts or interferes with something you eat or

drink. *For example, drinking grapefruit juice while taking certain medications may increase blood levels of these medicines.*

3. Drug-disease interactions: When a prescription or OTC medication interacts or interferes with a disease you have, you may experience a drug-disease interaction. *For example, decongestants, found in many cold remedies may cause your blood pressure to rise. This can be dangerous for individuals with hypertension.*

Instructions to prevent or reduce the risk of any of drug interactions: there are a few simple steps consumers can do to protect their health and avoid serious problems:

1. Read the label of all OTCs. Primarily, look for the section called "Drug Interactions Precaution." *Take only the recommended dose.*
2. Tell all of the doctors and pharmacists you visit about all of the prescription medications *and* OTC medicines you use. (Use the medication record in APPENDIX C or another acceptable form which can be found in materials suggested in the "Resources" section) Share your medication record with your doctor(s) and pharmacist(s) each time you see them.
3. Before taking any new medication, talk to your pharmacist or doctor. Make sure to talk about combining medicines (either prescription drugs or more than one OTC at a time). Ask if there are any foods, drinks, or medications you should avoid while taking the new OTC medicine.
4. Ask your doctor or pharmacist for advice on over-the-counter medicines.[5]

Rx to OTC Switches

There are two ways that prescription drugs become OTC: 1) drug review and 2) by a manufacturer's submission of additional information to the original drug application.

Currently, the FDA has stated that it will encourage more switches from Rx to OTC, by declaring a product "suitable" for nonprescription use. However, at this time, the FDA is not yet ready to orchestrate "forced switches" which would require Big Pharma to switch costly prescription drugs to OTC status once the FDA has determined that they are safe.

OTC Abuse

There have many cases of OTC abuse in the last few years. OTCS are generally safe, if taken as directed. But there are as many as 140 OTCs that contain an active ingredient that, if taken in large amounts, *can become dangerous and even deadly*. The National Institute for Drug Abuse is now listing this ingredient as a hallucinogen. The ingredient is not being identified here so as not to increase the widespread problem of abuse by young, impressionable teens discovering the accessibility of these drugs. Anyone with children should ask his or her physician or pharmacist for the names of *all* OTC medicines that have the potential for abuse.

In addition, there are some OTCs that contain an active ingredient that is used to create home-cooked, illegal methamphetamine-a powerful, addictive stimulant that enhances mood and body movement. There is now a movement by legislators as well as pharmacies to keep these OTCs behind-the-counter to limit the amount sold. (See the Chapter 18 for more information on behind-the-counter medications). In addition, individual states are seeking legislation to limit the accessibility of these OTC drugs. (Oklahoma was the first.)

The cost of OTCs

Most OTCs are less expensive than prescription drugs; however "the effect on consumers is mixed." This is because once a prescription drug becomes an OTC drug, 46% of American consumers who have prescription benefits are then required to pay *100%* of the cost instead of just a small percentage in the form of a copay or co-insurance. This is the primary reason for the concern by Consumer Groups when prescription drugs are switched to OTCs. Often, the "cost-shifting" not only impacts the one drug, but other drugs in the same therapeutic class. Americans *without* insurance, conversely, often benefit when a drug switches to OTC status, since they usually pay full retail price all the time anyway and OTCs are usually less expensive than the prescription version. In addition, consumers may also realize savings from eliminating a physician office visit, which is required for every new prescription drug.

Healthcare plans and insurers are delighted with "OTC switches" because they are no longer forced to pay the billions of dollars in sales for these blockbuster drugs. The ideal scenario would, of course, be that these savings would be passed on to the consumers or even the employers. However, more often than not, the savings are passed on to the

Relative Costs- Brand OTC vs. Generic vs. OTC	Cost
Average costs for OTC drugs in 2003 (*although usually not a 30 day supply*)	$7-$20
Average costs of a generic Rx in 2003	$28.74
Average Costs of a brand name Rx in 2003	$96.01
Average Cost of a co-pay for 30 day supply	$10-$30

healthcare plans, insurers, or PBMs.

The table below illustrates the differences in the cost between OTCs and prescription drugs in 2003:

However, this price comparison just doesn't tell the whole story. The OTC product sold in the store usually contains fewer doses than the previous prescription (e.g. not a 30 day supply), and most prescriptions,

Relative Costs- Brand Prilosec vs. Generic Prilosec (Omeprazole)v s. OTC—Prilosec	Brand Price Brand Copay 30 days-	Generic Price Generic Copay 30 days	OTC Price *28 days* 1 pill per day
Prilosec (Omeprazole) 20 mg. (*Not*-sustained release)	**$117!-** **$3.90** per dose	**$32.99** **$1.09** per dose **34 cents** per dose if paying copay	**$19.99** **71 cents** per dose

whether generic or brand Rx, will usually be at least a 30-day supply. To really compare prices, consumers need to compare the actual price per pill or per dose. For example, see the Prilosec prices below:

Clearly, the best value for the co*nsumer with prescription drug coverage* is a *generic version* of Prilosec, (not Prilosec *OTC*) because he can pay just a $10 copay (or 34 cents per dose!)

Comparison Shopping for OTCs

Like prescription drugs, it can be worth the reader's time to comparison shop for OTC drugs. OTC medicines, even more than prescription drugs, lend themselves to comparison-shopping; since they don't require a prescription and can be purchased almost anywhere. Savings can be found at local pharmacies or grocery stores, especially when products are on sale. OTCs can also be purchased in large quantities for an even better value at mass merchandising stores such as Costco. In addition, consumers can obtain *coupons* for OTC products right at the stores or on the Internet.

The Prilosec Story

Picture a fleet of 850 Proctor & Gamble Co. (P & G) delivery trucks rolling out to distribute Prilosec simultaneously to stores nationwide. This is exactly what P & G did on September 15, 2003 just after midnight, as part of a $100 million marketing campaign. As the trucks rolled out, so did the broadcast, print and billboard ads. The marketing campaign also included a traveling purple van driving through 24 cities in a "Burntown Challenge" Promotion.[6] The Prilosec "OTC switch" became a bona fide event and everywhere consumers went, there were Prilosec coupons and displays at grocery stores and pharmacies.

Prilosec OTC is part of a crowded market for the drug class known as proton-pump inhibitors, or PPIs. In 2001, Prilosec was the world's second largest selling drug, with *global* revenues of $5.7 billion. U.S. sales totaled $3.7 billion that year! Other branded versions on the market include Prevacid and Nexium (Nexium has the same active ingredient as Prilosec!) Although Prilosec OTC is available, prescription-strength

Prilosec will still be available for the foreseeable future for treating diseases that require diagnosis, such as ulcers and gastroesophageal reflux disease.

Incidentally, Prilosec, which has been known as the "little purple pill" is now *pink*-the pink color, is from the magnesium salt used to make the tablets.

Consumer Information

There are many excellent consumer brochures about OTCs. Some of the best include:

Brochure: *"Over-the-counter medicines: What's right for you?"* U.S. Food and Drug Administration and Consumer Healthcare Products Association. Rockville, MD. 2003. Available at http://www.fda.gov/cder/consumerinfo/WhatsRightForYou.htm
Handout: *"What you should Know About Over-the-Counter Medicines and Drug Interactions."* American Pharmacists Association. Available at www.pharmacyandyou.org.
Brochures: National Council on Patient Information and Education (NCPIE). 2004. Available at www.talkaboutrx.com

Conclusion

Overall, OTC drug products provide access and affordability for many wonderful medicines. In addition, they allow Americans to be involved in their own healthcare and empower them in many area of treatment where they usually feel helpless and vulnerable. However, consumers should remember that there are risks involved with OTC medications, as with any medications and they should always read the OTC labels and follow directions for use *to the letter.* Also, all OTC medicines should be added to your medication list (see APPENDIX C).

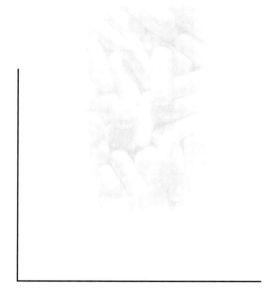

PART II: **BUYING PRESCRIPTION DRUGS IN THE <u>U.S.</u>**

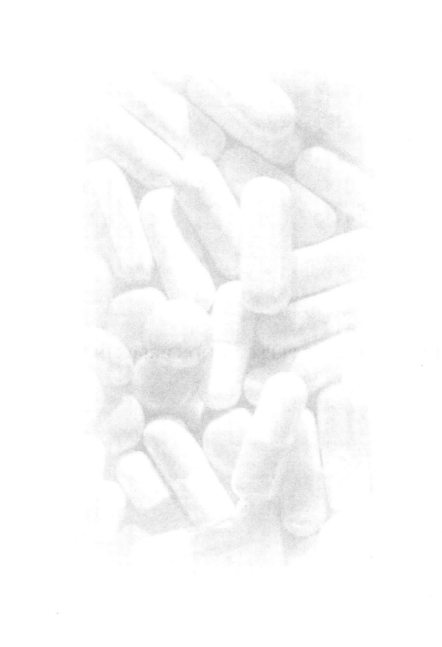

Chapter 11

Buying Prescription Drugs from <u>U.S.</u> Pharmacies

> **TIP:** Do some comparison-shopping before you actually need to buy prescription drugs. Find a pharmacist/ pharmacy you trust and that will provide discounts and stick with it!

Introduction

There are more than 50,000 pharmacies nationwide; nearly 15 million consumers pass through a retail pharmacy every day.[1] In fact, it seems like a new chain drugstore is popping up on almost every major intersection across the country, with many of them open 24 hours a day. Independent pharmacies are also alive and well. Interestingly enough, "independent pharmacies," which were edging toward extinction a few years ago, won top honors from *CONSUMER REPORTS* readers, besting the chains by an eye-popping margin. More than 85% of customers at independent drugstores were very satisfied or completely satisfied with their experience, compared with 58% of chain-drugstore customers."[2]

At the time this book was published, buying Prescription Drugs from U.S. pharmacies, either at stores or online, was still the best and only *legal* choice. However, this still leaves Americans with a wide array of options. Today, there are basically three types of U.S. pharmacies:

1. **Brick and Mortar Pharmacies**: This is a common term for pharmacies that are located in stores and have a walk-in presence. This includes pharmacies in grocery stores (e.g. Osco Drug in Albertsons stores), chain-drug stores (e.g. Walgreens), discount stores (e.g. Target), independent drug stores, (e.g. Medicine Shoppe) and mass merchandisers (e.g. Costco). Using brick and mortar pharmacies is still the most common method for purchasing prescriptions and arguably still the best. This is primarily due to convenience as well the patient/consumer counseling available

to individuals by the pharmacist(s) right at the store. If an individual knows his or her pharmacist by name and has built a good relationship with that pharmacist, then patient counseling is more likely to occur. The pharmacist also has knowledge of a patient's history, including what other drugs an individual is taking. This permits the pharmacist to screen for drug interactions and possible contraindications. NEVER UNDERESTIMATE THE IMPORTANCE OF THE PHARMACIST-PATIENT RELATIONSHIP.

2. **Internet and Online Pharmacies:** Internet pharmacies are businesses that sell prescription drugs (and other pharmacy products) via the Internet and then send the drug products to the consumers through the mail. They are also known as pharmacy intermediaries and most fill orders through arrangements with brick and mortar pharmacies. Examples include Drugstore.com and Discount Generics.US.

3. **"Brick and Clicks":** This is a term used to describe pharmacies that have *both* storefront *and* an on-line/Internet pharmacy options. Bricks and Clicks also frequently offer mail order, which may allow consumers to purchase 3-month supplies at a further reduced rate. Examples include Costco, CVS, and Target.

All three options have advantages, although clearly the "Bricks and Clicks" offer the widest range of services. All have bargain-hunting, comparison-shopping potential; however, it's recommended that each individual decide on <u>one pharmacy option and then stick with it.</u>

Tips for buying from U.S. pharmacies

There are many ways to save money when buying prescription drugs from U.S. pharmacies. The goal is to *never* pay full retail, especially on *brand name* prescription drugs.

Cost saving strategies includes:

Shop Around: If readers had the opportunity to call several pharmacies in their area, they would discover that prescription drug prices can vary as much as *10-40% or more* from location to location. Even with that substantial difference, if a consumer purchases only 1-3 *prescription* drugs a year, it probably is *not* worth the extra effort to shop around. However, if the consumer is one of many Americans who spend over $*1,400* a year, 10-40% can make a big difference in an annual household budget. APPENDIX D contains a cost comparison tool to help readers determine if shopping around will be worth it. Once that decision is made, it is recommended that the readers (and their families) find a "pharmacy home" and put down "roots," at least for all prescription drug purchases. Shopping around for *OTC* bargains may also be worthwhile, once a consumer has had the initial counseling for the OTC drug(s) and has added the OTCs to their Medication Record (see APPENDIX C).

When shopping around, readers may want to: 1) check APPENDIX A for price comparisons, and 2) telephone the individual pharmacies and/or check prices on the Internet. Two great websites to use to check prices include: www.pricescan.com or the author's website: www.prescriptionpathway.com. However, be advised that these sites are not *State* specific. Specific statewide pricing may often be available through the individual State Prescription Assistance Program or through the individual State Attorney General's office. For those individuals who live in a state where pharmacies are required to produce a prescription drug price list, *ask for the list* (e.g. New York).

NOTE: Please be advised that, although comparison-shopping for prescription drugs may be recommended in this book, it should never be undertaken lightly. Prescription drugs are *not* avocados or automobiles, and patient counseling and prescription drug review are important components of the purchasing process. It is also recommended that comparison-shopping be done *prior* to the actual need for a prescription drug so that the process can be studied and the strategy chosen, based not only on price, but on the availability and accessibility of a qualified, trusted pharmacist.

Once a consumer picks a pharmacy, he or she should *stick* with that pharmacy, whenever possible.

Consider using a Mass Merchandiser such as Costco Wholesale or Sam's Club: If only one recommendation could be made in this book for *where* to purchase prescription drugs, this would be it. Although warehouse club/mass merchandiser stores are not available in every city, there are more than 650 of them in the U.S. Additionally, even when there is *not* a mass merchandiser store available in the area, consumers can still participate in their mail order programs. *Many* of the cost-saving strategies listed in this chapter can be utilized at these pharmacies.

Advantages of using pharmacies such as Costco include:
1. <u>ALL</u> prescription drugs are automatically discounted. There is no need to wonder if a drug is on a "formulary," included on a "discount card" or subject to drastic price fluctuations.
2. Consumers have the choice of both a brick-and-mortar store *and* mail order pharmacy.
3. *Everyone* receives a discount-there are no eligibility or enrollment requirements.
4. CONSUMERS DO <u>NOT</u> NEED TO BUY A CLUB MEMBERSHIP TO SHOP AT THE PHARMACY BECAUSE PRESCRIPTION DRUGS ARE FEDERALLY REGULATED. If a consumer is only purchasing prescription drugs, a club membership card is <u>not</u> needed; the consumer needs only to tell the assistant at the door that he or she is dropping off or picking up a prescription. Consumers can then walk right in (and use the pharmacy only). The author has tested this at least a dozen times at a local Costco and never had a problem.

Costco is the author's **#1 choice** (among mass merchants, as well as other pharmacies),because they post their prices on the Internet, which makes comparison-shopping much easier. They also have superior service and great prices.

Ask for Generics: In the U.S., generics are still the very best buy. Consumers/patients should always ask their physician and/or pharmacist if they are receiving a generic and if not, why not. If there is *no* generic available, it's worth asking the physician if there *is* a generic drug available *in the same therapeutic class* that's as effective and as well tolerated. Sometimes there will be a good alternative, sometimes not. (See Chapter 4 for more information about generic prescription drugs.)

Ask for Drug Samples or Drug Coupons: If the physician is prescribing an expensive brand- name drug because it is the best treatment option, then patients should ask the physician for drug samples. Drug samples, as discussed in Chapter 5, are packages of a 1 week to 1month supply of brand name drugs given to the physicians by the drug companies to give to their patients.

Drug samples benefit needy patients without insurance, allow patients to try a drug to see if it can be tolerated, and also allow doctors to gain early experience with new medicines. Drug samples may not always be available; however, it doesn't hurt to ask.

Drug coupons are provided by the drug company and are available in pharmacies and/or the drug companies' websites. The coupons are usually good for just a 7-day supply, but it's still often long enough for a patient to see if he or she can tolerate the drug before a further investment is made. Examples of websites with coupons include: www.celebrex.com. www.lipitor.com, www.purplepill.com (Nexium), etc. (Note: when printing a coupon directly from a website, be aware that if a pop-up blocker is "on" at the computer being used, it may block the coupon as it is popping up and usually there are *no second chances* to ask for another coupon.) Also,

BE ADVISED that you will need <u>two</u> separate prescription forms: one for the drug coupon supply and one for a regular 30-90 day supply.

Use Mail order for maintenance drugs for chronic conditions: Mail order has become increasingly popular over the last few years, with sales rising to $32.5 billion.[3] Mail order is a great option for consumers who are part of a "group." For example, someone with prescription drug benefits through his or her employer is part of a "group." Mail order is also offered through drug discount card programs (See chapter 7) and managed by Pharmacy Benefits Managers (PBMs). In addition, some brick and click pharmacies like Costco and Target, as well as all the U.S. Internet pharmacies, offer mail order. With mail order, consumers can purchase optimum quantities (usually a 3-month supply) of chronic medications via mail, fax, telephone, email, or the Internet. The primary advantages to mail order are:

1) Cost savings-only <u>one</u> copay is charged instead of three. In addition, the mail order prices are often better than in-store prices.
2) Convenience- no trip to the store.
3) Additional services- mail order programs offer prescription management, disease management and patient compliance programs.

Note: One hassle: Most state pharmacy laws will not allow a *copy* of a prescription to be faxed or mailed by a consumer, so the <u>*original*</u> prescription form will need to be mailed, or a telephone call made by the prescribing physician. Sometimes this can be a major inconvenience. Consumers should *always* make a copy of the prescription form for their records prior to mailing the original in case it gets lost or in case the mail order company has questions.

Purchase in "Ideal Quantities": "Ideal quantity" and "optimum quantity" are terms used to denote the *largest number of unit doses* that a patient can purchase with a single prescription. The actual number varies and is based on the drug's effectiveness, side effects, costs, and/or insurance. A 3-month supply is the most common ideal quantity, although 6-months may be acceptable and may offer additional savings. Purchasing in "ideal quantities" or bulk, as some call it, is one of the best cost-savings strategies; the prices are lower per unit dose and the number of copays required is reduced. Consumers who purchase chronic medications should always purchase in "ideal quantities." The only exception might be when a physician has prescribed a new drug; a 30-day supply would give a patient a chance to determine if a drug is effective and well tolerated before paying for a greater number of pills.

Consider Using Discount Cards: As discussed in Chapter 7, a prescription drug discount card provides small discounts on prescription drugs and is a viable option for some groups of people. Although the savings may only be 10-20%, this is still preferable to paying full retail. Examples of groups that may benefit by the use of discount cards are Medicare recipients and consumers who live in smaller towns who don't have access to pharmacies that provide discounts such as Costco. For Medicare recipients, a quick price comparison can be done using the www.medicare.gov website.

Purchase chronic medications from Internet websites, preferably the Brick and Click: This is a recommendation that combines the "mail order" strategy with the "ideal quantity" strategy. Some U.S. Internet pharmacy prices are very similar to Costco prices. For more information on U.S. Internet pharmacies, see Chapter 12.

Determine if OTCs are an option: As discussed in Chapter 10, oftentimes OTC drugs can be a less expensive option over more costly prescription drugs for certain chronic conditions. An obvious example is using Aspirin or Motrin (to treat arthritis) vs. Vioxx or Celebrex. In addition, a physician office visit is not required for "refills" which may provide additional savings. However, this cost-savings strategy should never be used without a physician's approval. As discussed in Chapter 10, generic or store brand OTCs are usually less expensive than brand name OTCs.

Purchase prescription drugs with $10 copays whenever possible: For patients with prescription drug coverage and a 3-tier copay system, purchasing generics or other Tier 1 prescription drugs will also provide a cost-savings. The difference between $10 and $30 can really add up, especially for consumers who take a lot of chronic medications. Consumers with prescription drug coverage should consider taking a copy of the drug formulary to all physician office visits. By the time a consumer arrives at a pharmacy, he or she should already know if the drug is covered, under what 'tier' the drug is classified, and what the copay will be.

Ask your physician if "pill splitting" is permitted: "Pill splitting" is the controversial practice of cutting or splitting a tablet of a higher dose in order to save money. Splitting a pill in half can sometimes give two pills for the price of one because many times the prices are the same or nearly the same for two different strengths (e.g. 20 mg. and 40 mg.) This only works on some tablets and not on capsules or time-released formulations.

Some healthcare plans and organizations are advocating pill splitting as a cost savings strategy. The list of prescription drugs that qualify for pill splitting is limited. A study conducted by Stanford School of Medicine researchers started with 265 medications and eventually came up with a list of 11 common medications that qualified for pill splitting.[4] Cost savings for these 11 drugs ranged from 23%-50%. The 11 prescription drugs were:

Cardura	Klonopin	Paxil
Celexa	Serzone	Pravachol
Lipitor	Viagra	Zestril
Zoloft	Zyprexa	

This practice, as controversial as it is, should not be undertaken without a physician's approval. Some consumers, especially the elderly, have problems with splitting the pill accurately, even when it's a scored tablet. A good quality plastic pill splitter should be purchased (and can be purchased for under $7). A pharmacist may offer to do the job, but this is rare. Consumers should also split the pills as soon as they purchase them so they don't forget and accidentally take the wrong dose.

Ask the pharmacy for a "price match": Many pharmacies have stated that they will match other pharmacy prices. This may or may not actually be the case. Smaller independent pharmacies are more likely to honor a price match than a chain pharmacy because they have more control over their prices.

Explore Patient Assistance Programs: Patient Assistance Programs, (PAPs), are an excellent source of free or low-cost prescription drugs for those meeting the income requirements. For more information on PAPs, see Chapter 9.

Use reliable websites for "price checks": This book is a great place to start to check prices (See APPENDIX A), but actual prices will fluctuate and become out-of-date. There are several websites that provide very good information on current prescription drug prices. In other words, "let your fingers do the walking." Valuable websites include, but are not limited to:

www.CRBestBuyDrugs.org: Provides national price averages on prescription drugs in specific drug classes (e.g. cholesterol lowering drugs). Evidence-based research on the efficacy and safety of the drugs are also included.

www.medicare.gov: Provides comparison prices for all of the Medicare discount cards. Hopefully, after January 2006, the website will provide a comparison of prices for plans participating in the new Medicare Part D.

www.costco.com: Provides prices on prescription drugs for only Costco, but the prices are *very* good. Costco has both brick-and-mortar stores as well as a mail order option.

www.destinationrx.com: Searches for deals from a variety of online U.S. pharmacies.

www.pharmacychecker.com: Provides prices for a variety of foreign and U.S. pharmacies. This is a good site because the pharmacies must meet certain criteria in order to be listed as a participatory pharmacy or pharmacy intermediary.

www.pricescan.com: Provides prices for a variety of foreign and U.S. pharmacies.

In addition, readers should check the author's website: **www.prescription-pathway.com** on a monthly basis. The author's website will continue to provide tips on comparison-shopping, as well as current prices for the top prescription drugs according to sales and volume.

Conclusion

In general, purchasing prescription drugs from U.S. Pharmacies is still the best option. Purchases can be made at brick and mortar stores or through U.S. Internet Pharmacies (For more on Internet pharmacies, see Chapter 12.) There are many cost-savings strategies that can provide 10-40% off of full retail prices. Some strategies require comparison-shopping; others require a dialogue with a patient's physician and/or pharmacist and a few are just common sense.

As discussed previously, after comparison-shopping, consumers should pick a pharmacy "home" and stick with it! This will ensure that all safety measures will be taken. It will also promote the development of a pharmacist-patient relationship.

Chapter 12
Buying Prescription Drugs from <u>U.S.</u> Internet Pharmacies

> **TIP: Always purchase your prescription drugs from reliable sources as listed in this book. Never trust a random Internet Ad received via E-mail or through pop-up ads.**

Introduction

Everyday we read about senior citizens and uninsured Americans buying prescriptions via the Internet. Surveys show that 9% of U.S. consumers who take prescription drugs purchase them online; this amounts to just 4% of Americans.[1] In addition, 7% of consumers have used the Internet to research drugs (7%) and another (5%) have used the Internet to find the best prescription drug prices. Three percent have gone online to order a drug, but picked it up offline.[2]

It's projected that there are thousands of websites that sell prescription drugs! Approximately 50% of these are U.S. websites and 50% are foreign websites. *In 2004, 19 million Americans purchased prescription drugs online from licensed U.S. pharmacies!*[3]

There are three types of Internet or online pharmacies, based on their purchasing policies. They are:
1. <u>Prescription</u>: Websites that require an *original* prescription form to be mailed or called in to the pharmacy.
2. <u>Online consultation:</u> Websites that conduct an online consultation, based on a questionnaire submitted by the consumer. They use a "physician" who is contracted with the pharmacy to write a prescription based on that completed questionnaire. *This violates many state pharmacy laws. Stay away from these sites!*
3. <u>No-prescription:</u> Websites that sell prescription drugs *without* a prescription from the patient's physician or *any* physician. *Stay away from these sites!*

Not all pharmacies offer all prescription drugs. Some offer a full-range,

some a partial range and some just offer lifestyle and/or 50 popular medications. Most of the reputable sites will offer all the common prescription drugs.

Purchasing prescription drugs via the Internet

PROS

1. It's easy. All a consumer needs to order drugs online is a credit
   card, a computer, and a phone line.
2. It may be cost-effective: Some Internet pharmacies (e.g. www.drug-
   store.com) may have better prices than the brick and mortar pharmacies because they have lower overhead costs and can buy in
   large volumes. Online pharmacies also allow consumers to comparison-shop for the best prices since their prices are posted on
   the Internet. Some of them even accept healthcare plans (insurance) and discount cards (e.g. Drugstore.com).
3. It affords privacy and anonymity: Some customers may feel more
   comfortable purchasing drugs or asking questions by phone or
   online than they would in person at a walk-in pharmacy in their
   neighborhood.
4. It may be convenient: For people who find it physically difficult
   to travel to a local pharmacy or for those who live in rural areas,
   it may be more convenient to use online pharmacies.
5. It's legal: Unlike buying from *foreign* Internet websites, buying
   prescription drugs from *U.S.* Internet pharmacies is legal in most
   cases. However, it's only legal if the online pharmacy doesn't
   violate any state pharmacy laws or U.S. postal service laws. In
   addition, Internet pharmacies must require a valid prescription for
   prescription drugs and must have current state licenses for both
   the pharmacy as well as the pharmacists themselves. A consumer
   can take legal action more readily if something goes wrong when
   U.S. laws govern the websites.
6. It provides additional services: In order to be competitive, many
   online pharmacies have added extra services- Services allow consumers to: 1) E-mail questions to pharmacists 24/7, 2) research
   medical topics, 3) search online for potentially dangerous drug

interactions, and 4) receive e-mail reminders. In addition, some Internet companies such as Drugstore.com will also alert clients if the branded drug they are taking becomes available in generic form. However, readers should know that brick and mortar pharmacies offer many of these services as well.

CONS

1. It *might* be unsafe: There are real safety concerns when buying prescription drugs online and Americans are wise to be cautious. Caution and knowledge are without a doubt the best lines of defense. One current study of consumers showed that 60% of adults think drugs bought on the Internet are not as safe as those bought from a drugstore. Some U.S. pharmacies are *not* licensed, provide *no* security of protected health information, *no* security for credit card information, and provide *no* counseling or contact information. To minimize these risks, consumers should buy only from the best (see guidelines below).

2. It can be difficult to get the exact number of doses: This may include the inability to fill any and all quantities (For example, if a patient has a prescription for 35 pills, an Internet pharmacy may only have 30, 90 or 100 day quantities available and therefore cannot fill that specific prescription.) Sometimes there are additional fees such as medical fees, shipping fees and account setup fees when purchasing online.

3. It's too easy to purchase drugs with the potential of abuse: With both legitimate and illegitimate U.S. Internet pharmacies, it's easy to see why obtaining *all types* of drugs online is far too easy. This includes drugs that are controlled substances with high risks of addiction and drug complications. The U.S. government and other interested parties are trying to implement solutions to curtail this problem, but with the Internet so accessible, any member of the family can find a way to purchase drugs online with a credit card. Parents should always closely monitor credit card purchases.

4. <u>Privacy can be compromised by sharing information with third parties:</u> Disreputable sites will share personal and health information with marketing companies and even pornography sites. Spam is a real problem and companies can make big profits from selling e-mail lists.

5. <u>Consumers purchasing goods over the Internet are required by law to pay appropriate state and local sales taxes.</u> Taxpayers are supposed to be responsible for determining the amounts of local taxes they need to pay from online purchases and to send a check to their governments each year! Many consumers are not aware of this and even when they are, most people are non-compliant.

Caution: 10 pharmaceuticals <u>not</u> to be purchased via the Internet

The FDA has singled out 10 popular pharmaceuticals that should <u>not</u> be purchased via the Internet or from foreign sources because of the risks involved with their use. They include:[5]

1. Accutane: an acne treatment
2. Actiq: for management of severe cancer pain
3. Clozaril: a schizophrenia drug
4. Lotronex: for irritable bowel syndrome in women
5. Mifeprex (or RU-486):   for the termination of early intrauterine pregnancy
6. Thalomid: for treatment of erythema nodosum leprosum
7. Tikosyn: a sinus drug
8. Tracleer: for pulmonary arterial hypertension
9. Trovan: for severe, life threatening disease
10. Zyrem: for the treatment of cataplexy in narcolepsy patients

<u>Consumers should never purchase any of these prescription drugs from any foreign or domestic Internet websites</u>. If a reader identifies any of them as a drug purchased online, he/she should talk to his physicians as soon as possible!

Guidelines for buying prescription drugs from U.S. Internet sites

Caution is required when purchasing prescription drugs from U.S. Internet sites, but the benefits can be well worth it. The following guidelines are suggested:

1. <u>Buy from VIPPS Internet websites</u>: In 1999, the National Association Boards of Pharmacy implemented the Verified Internet Pharmacy Practice Sites ™ (VIPPS®) program. The VIPPS seal of approval identifies to the public the online pharmacy practice websites that are appropriately licensed, legitimately operating via the Internet and those that have successfully completed a rigorous criteria review and inspection. Currently, there are only approximately 13 companies licensed by VIPPS and since it is a *voluntary* program, it does not include all credible "bricks and clicks." In fact, some of the best 'bricks and clicks' are *not* certified. VIPPS certification is more essential for companies that are Internet pharmacies only. For further information, readers should visit the website: <u>www.nabp.net/vipps</u>.

2. <u>Verify that State Pharmacy Boards license the Internet pharmacies:</u> The individual States Boards of Pharmacy have primary responsibility for regulation of online pharmacies. The state board of pharmacy in which the pharmacy is physically located mainly exercises regulatory authority. In addition, most states protect their citizens by licensing out-of-state pharmacies that ship medications to patients in their jurisdictions. Readers can check the National Association of Board Pharmacies for license verification at: <u>www.nabp.net</u>.

3. <u>Review the 'ratings' for U.S. Internet Pharmacies</u> at <u>www.pharmacychecker.com.</u> Pharmacychecker.com is a for-profit company that conducts reviews for both foreign and U.S. online pharmacies and evaluates them based on 5 criteria: 1) pharmacy licensure 2) SSL encryptions for financial transactions 3) privacy policy 4) prescription requirement and 5) contact information. For more information on Pharmacychecker.com, see Chapter 13.

4. <u>Check to see if the U.S. Internet site accepts healthcare plans/ insurance.</u> If a reader has prescription drug coverage through a healthcare plan, he or she can still utilize many Internet pharmacies; however, not *all* sites accept all insurance. For example, Drugstore.com and Costco.com accept many healthcare plans. Readers should verify coverage *prior* to purchasing from the online pharmacy in order to prevent complications later.

5. <u>Check to see if there are additional fees for shipping and handling, etc.</u> The savings may not be as substantial once all the fees are added in. In a recent survey, 35% of respondents stated that surprise costs would lead them to abandon a purchase online.[4] Some of the best websites such as <u>www.drugstore.com</u> and <u>www.costo.com</u> do *not* charge shipping and handling; however, this should be explored *prior* to choosing the online pharmacy.

6. <u>Choose a pharmacy that offers free phone consultation with a pharmacist and free ask-a-pharmacist E-mail service,</u> When possible, a consumer should establish a relationship with a pharmacist at an online pharmacy, just as he or she would with a pharmacist at a brick and mortar pharmacy. The free consultation and E-mail service are usually the only links a consumer has with actual people who work at the pharmacy.

7. <u>Consider choosing a "brick and click"- they are still your best option and offer the best flexibility.</u> If a consumer chooses a pharmacy that operates only online and problems arise, it can be a major hassle to receive timely resolutions. With online pharmacies that also have a brick and mortar site, patients can always go to that pharmacy's store as a back up.

8. <u>Be aware that generally, in order to be valid, state laws require faxed prescriptions to be received directly from the prescriber (e.g. physician) and **not** the patient.</u> Patients *must* obtain an original prescription from their physician, preferably for the "optimum quantity" and then either mail it, or have the physician mail it or fax it to the online pharmacy. Patients should *always* keep a copy of the prescription form in case the original gets lost in the mail. In addition, when the prescription drugs are received via

mail, patients can then check the name on the bottle with the name on the copy of the prescription form to verify that they received the correct drug.

FDA Guidelines for websites

The FDA has created the following guidelines or tips to help consumers protect themselves when they buy medications online:
1. Require a prescription from the patient's doctor or other health care professional who is licensed in the U.S. to write prescriptions for that patient for that medicine.
2. Check each prescription. Look for a policy on the website that tells you how the prescription will be checked.
3. Have a licensed pharmacist answer your questions.
4. Have a way for consumers to talk to a real person if there are problems.

Conclusion

Buying prescriptions online from a reputable U.S. Internet pharmacy can be a very satisfactory experience. It can also provide substantial cost savings for consumers who must purchase many brand name drugs. In Chapter 16, where "Prescription Pathways" are presented to save consumers money, readers will find U.S. Internet pharmacies listed as a preferred choice. The author recommends www.costco.com and www.drugstore.com.

PART III: BUYING PRESCRIPTION DRUGS IN THE <u>CANADA</u>

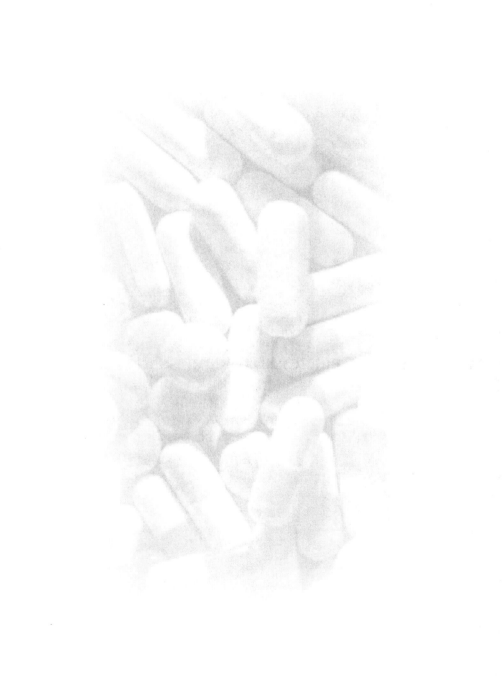

Chapter 13
What's in store if you buy from Canada?

> **TIP:** Do your research before deciding on this option. First, check out Prescription Pathways in Chapter 16 and then use the Cost Savings worksheet in APPENDIX D to determine if it's really worth it to buy from Canada. If you do, use all safety precautions.

Meet Mrs. Jones, an unassuming 70-year-old American bargain hunter. She is one of over 1 million Americans who purchase their prescription drugs from Canada. Mrs. Jones, like many of the elderly, takes brand name prescription drugs for chronic conditions such as high cholesterol, high blood pressure, diabetes, and osteoarthritis. While most Americans are buying their prescription drugs at local pharmacies, Mrs. Jones and other seniors are hopping on board a bus every few months and traveling to Canada where the top 10 brand- name prescription drugs are often 30% less expensive than in the U.S. Currently, Mrs. Jones can save up to $1,600 per year by buying from Canada!

Introduction

Stories like Mrs. Jones's have been dominating the front page of newspapers and magazines for years. This is due to the fact that the sick and elderly are one of America's most vulnerable populations with at least one-third of their number having no prescription coverage. The elderly and disabled also use the greatest number of prescription drugs. If there is truly a healthcare crisis and a crisis of cost, conscience and availability of prescription drugs, the seniors and the disabled are definitely the moving targets.

Seniors, advocacy organizations, and state and local governments are making news by fighting back *on their own terms* against Big Pharma and bloated U.S. brand name drug prices. One way they are doing this is by purchasing prescription drugs from Canada and other countries.

The practice of buying prescription drugs from Canada has continued to increase and to some, it's rising at an alarming rate. Consider:

1. In 2003, Americans imported more than $<u>1.4 billion</u> in prescription drugs. (Note: Although this sounds like a lot, this is still *less than 1%* of the total U.S. prescription drug sales.)
2. Approximately one-half or $700 million of the prescription drug imports in 2003 (via mail) came from Canada.
3. Nearly *two million* Americans order prescription drugs from Canada each year.
4. Approximately *20 million* packages of drugs per year enter the U.S. illegally through the *mail* system and about half of them are from Canadian pharmacies.
5. Many prescription drugs enter the country via a "land border." Approximately 25,000 to 30,000 Americans walk across an international bridge (into many different countries) on a daily basis.
6. While the exact *number* of *prescriptions* entering the U.S. from Canada via foot traffic is unknown, the value is estimated at an additional $500 million a year;
7. Canada remains the most popular foreign location for drug reimportation due to safety and convenience.

Not only are individuals and busloads of seniors buying from Canada, *but also city, county, and state governments are following suit.* As this practice continues to be more pervasive, readers need a source to obtain accurate information about purchasing drugs from Canada. This is why this book is important and why the author believes in further open discussions about reimportation.

Consider that:

- Some physicians who live in towns near a Canadian border town now often have licenses to prescribe prescription drugs in *both* countries.
- Studies show that approximately 45% of Americans don't even realize that the practice of buying prescription drugs from Canada is illegal.

- Some Canadian pharmacies in border towns may have more

than 100,000 clients, with the majority of them living in the U.S.

- City and state governments have been able to demonstrate substantial savings for their governments when allowing employees to purchase prescription drugs from Canada.

Cost savings

So how substantial *are* the savings and is Mrs. Jones's experience atypical? A study by the American Association of Retired Persons (AARP) printed in April 2003 showed savings of between 46 *and 52%* on six commonly prescribed drugs. *As of 2005, however, the savings are probably closer to 25-30%, due to many factors, including a stronger Canadian dollar.*

The table below shows price comparisons for 12 commonly prescribed *brand* name prescription drugs from both a U.S. online pharmacy and a Canadian online pharmacy in 2005:

Name and dose of drugs 30 or 90-day supply	U.S. Price	Canadian Price
Lipitor 20 mg.	$275.97 for 90	$199.36 for 100
Zocor 20 mg.	$356.97 for 90	$222.87 for 100
Prevacid 15 mg.	$ 77.17 for 30	$66.74 for 30
Propecia 1 mg.	$49.99 for 30	$44.16 for 28
Zyprexa 10 mg.	$559.99 for 90	$494.75 for 100
Zoloft 50 mg.	$209.97for 100	$172.50 for 100
Celebrex 200 mg.	$213.99 for 90	$133.49 for 100
Neurontin 100 mg.	$45.99 for 90	$46.27 for 100
Norvasc 5 mg.	$123.97 for 90	$124.55 for 100
Pravachol 20 mg.	$87.99 for 30	$64.84 for 30
Fosamax 10 mg.	$72.99 for 30	$61.73 for 30
Singulair 10 mg.	$89.99 for 30	$65.99 for 30

Note:
Prices were effective 4/05. For more information, see Appendix A.

Substantial Cost savings- The "Hot List"

In fact, savings will probably not be substantial enough to be worth the risks and hassle of buying prescriptions drugs in Canada, *unless* individuals are purchasing costly *brand name* drugs.

Brand name drugs that might provide a substantial savings include those listed in the table below. The author calls this the "Hot List." **If a reader has not been prescribed two or more of the brand name drugs listed below, then there is probably not enough of a savings to buy from Canada:**

Allegra	Aricept	Clarinex
Celebrex	Celexa	Crestor
Effexor XR	Flonase	Glucophage XL
Lipitor	Lopressor	Nexium
Nasonex	Ortho Evra	Paxil CR
Plavix	Pravachol	Prevacid
Procrit	Risperdal	Synthroid
Viagra	Risperdal	Singulair
Zyrtec	Zocor	Zoloft
Zetia	Zyprexa	Depakote

(For an updated "Hot List," see wwww.prescriptionpathway.com.)

Why it costs less in Canada

Prices are usually less expensive in Canada for *Americans* for the following reasons:

    a. <u>Price Controls-</u> In Canada, a government review board sets the prices of *new* brand name drugs and limits the increases on *existing* brand name drugs to no more than inflation. Due to price controls, the drug companies are not allowed to gouge consumers for new brand name drugs and therefore the *difference* between the costs of brand name and generic drugs is minimal. However because generics and brand name drugs whose patents have expired are <u>not</u> regulated, *generic* prescription drugs in Canada are *more expensive* than generics in the U.S., often by as much as 50-70%! Just two generic drug companies in Canada control nearly 60% of the total market. Here is the irony: Canadians often buy their generics <u>from U.S.</u> mail order pharmacies! Another thought-provoking point: *U.S. pharmaceutical companies are required under a 1994 treaty to sell their drugs at drastically cut prices to countries with drug price controls.* Any pharmaceutical company that fails to comply risks losing its patent protection.

b. <u>The favorable dollar exchange rate</u>- Due to the U.S. dollar's strength relative to the Canadian dollar, Americans already have a built in discount of over 20%. Therefore, if the savings totals 40%, the dollar exchange rate accounts for approximately half the savings! For example, let's say that a 3-month supply of Lipitor costs $183.97 at <u>www.drugstore.com</u> (a U.S. Internet pharmacy). In Canada, the same Lipitor costs $206.22 *Canadian;* however, the exchange rate allows Americans to purchase Canadian Lipitor from a Canadian Internet pharmacy for $153.20 in *U.S. dollars, which is less than at the U.S. Internet pharmacy.*

c. <u>Drugs are developed in the U.S. so other countries don't have to bear the R & D costs</u>: This has long been a sore point for many Americans. The reason that prescription drugs cost U.S. consumers up to 3,000% more than the actual manufacturing costs is partially due to the fact that Americans are paying the brunt of the world's R & D, both for the drug they are purchasing, as well as for drugs yet to be developed. As discussed in Chapter 2, for every 5,000 treatments tested, only 5 make to clinical trials and then just 1 of the 5 ends up on drugstore shelves. However, the R & D objection may be flawed since a large portion of the NMEs (new medical entities) came from Europe in 2004. Both Europe and Asia have NMEs in the pipeline for the coming year.

d. <u>Canada caps the liabilities of drug companies</u>. The cap on malpractice and liability aids in keeping prescription drug prices lower in Canada.

How it works

To date, there are 4 basic ways to purchase drugs from Canada:

1. <u>Purchase from a land border in Canada:</u> A smaller portion of prescription drug sales from Canada are obtained through actual visits to a Canadian city, where the prescription drugs are bought then hand carried across a land border. Seniors may travel alone in individual cars, but usually prefer to go by organized busloads. This way there is a liaison present to explain the ins and outs of the process.

2. <u>Purchase from a Canadian Internet website</u>: This is the most popular method as well as the most convenient. There are at least 45 reputable Canadian Internet pharmacies/pharmacy intermediaries.

3. <u>Purchase through state, county, and local governments that have implemented Canadian purchasing programs</u>: Governments with tight budgets can save millions of dollars by permitting citizens to purchase prescription drugs from Canada. Some Americans see these government programs as progressive, but others see them as just illegal. There are over 12 city, county, and state governments who have implemented reimportation programs for government employees, seniors, the disabled, and/or the uninsured.

4. <u>Purchase from a storefront in the U.S. that serves as an intermediary to Canadian pharmacies</u>. Several for-profit companies have set up "storefronts" in malls and office buildings and act as intermediaries for U.S. consumers. Basically, consumers hand carry their prescriptions to the storefronts, make price comparisons, and then order their prescription drugs from Canada by using these intermediaries.

Is it safe?

Many consumers don't realize that in 2002, $40.7 billion of the prescription drugs taken by Americans were already imported from foreign countries! [1] This represented a nearly five-fold increase from $8.7 billion in 1995.[2] Seventeen of the 20 largest drug companies worldwide now manufacture drugs in Ireland. For example, Pfizer's Lipitor, the largest-selling drug in the world, is manufactured in Ireland. There are also manufacturing plants in Sweden, France, Japan and Singapore.[3] Although the *labeling and packaging requirements* are different for drugs destined for the U.S., the drugs are therapeutically the same, whether they are shipped to America or anywhere else in the world. The manufacturing plants must still meet all the FDA's good manufacturing practices during inspections, both before the initial plant opening and during periodic inspections. The primary difference in the case of importing the $40.7 billion is that *Big Pharma, and not individuals,* is the group doing the importing! In fact, some blame the pharmaceutical companies for the current trade deficit.

Many Americans are familiar with the study and the accompanying "raid" that was performed and publicized by the FDA in 2004 during a counterfeit drug crackdown. (This is also discussed in Chapter 3.) In the 3-day blitz, the FDA intercepted 1,982 packages from foreign and U.S. pharmacies at mail facilities and courier hubs in the U.S. The FDA stated that 1,178 of the drugs were "unapproved." Upon closer look, most were foreign generic versions of FDA-approved drugs and had packaging and handling problems; however, not one serious problem was identified from authentic, reputable Canadian pharmacies. In fact, only *Canadian* pharmacies consistently required a patient-provided prescription. Just five of the twenty-nine U.S. pharmacies could say the same.

TO THE AUTHOR'S KNOWLEDGE, as of the printing of this book, there have been <u>no</u> counterfeit, adulterated, or contaminated prescription drugs purchased by Americans from *authentic, reputable Canadian* pharmacies. The author knows of only **one** known case of counterfeit prescription drugs found at a Canadian pharmacy. In June 2005, counterfeit versions of Norvasc were found at a local pharmacy in Hamilton, Ontario. (The presumed fakes were grayish or beige in color, not white, and the writing of the NRV and number 10 on the pills were different.) This was the first seizure of its kind in the area, and possibly in Canada.

Additionally, there has been only one known recent case of a drug recall for a batch of Singulair; however, it was not related to tampering or counterfeiting.

Another point to consider when discussing the safety of drug importation is that Europe has been engaging in what is called "parallel trade" for years. This is the legal European practice of importing and exporting lower-cost drugs across 18 national borders. In Europe, where it is very well controlled, there have been no reports of counterfeiting. In fact, some think that this practice is probably safer than buying drugs from unknown sources on the Internet, because the prescription drugs are sold directly to the pharmacists or a pharmacy intermediary. (For more information on parallel trade see Chapter 14.)

U.S. regulators believe that allowing the importation of drugs from other countries would simply give counterfeiters the ability to contaminate the drug supply earlier in the process. This has *never* been proven, however.

Understanding Reimportation- IT'S ILLEGAL!

What is "Reimportation?"

In order to understand purchasing options from Canada, it's important for consumers to understand the concept of "reimportation." Reimportation is the term that was coined to describe the purchasing of prescription drugs from Canada and other foreign countries by Americans. Definitions include:

1. Importation: The practice of purchasing medications in another country or from a foreign Internet site that are *manufactured in another country* and then brought into the U.S. via the mail or carried across a land border. For example, a U.S. consumer purchases a Canadian generic version of Zoloft (Apo-sertraline) from a Canadian Internet website and the package is sent to the consumer's home.

2. Reimportation: The practice of purchasing medications *manufactured in the U.S.* and exported to a foreign country and then *brought back (reimported) into the U.S.* The term 'reimportation' is used incorrectly in most cases, because the drugs being purchased in Canada are not usually made here in the U.S but rather

are manufactured in Canada or Europe.

At the time of the publishing of this book, importation and reimportation of prescription drugs from other countries by anyone other than the original manufacturer *was still illegal.* And it was not just illegal according to federal statutes (i.e. the FDA). As of July 2005, purchasing prescription drugs from foreign pharmacies violated many state pharmacy laws, U.S. postal laws and U.S. customs laws.

However, the fact that it is illegal has *not* stopped individuals and groups from importing drugs from Canada. Seniors, state, county, and local governments, advocacy groups, and for-profit companies/storefronts are still importing prescription drugs and there is no reason to believe the practice will cease unless the cost savings cease. Senator Joe Lieberman described the trend of buying drugs from Canada as "a kind of Boston Tea Party of the 21st Century." The "court of public opinion" continues to weigh in as over 70% of Americans continue to approve of reimportation.

The FDA associate commissioner for Policy and Planning, William K. Hubbard stated: "Virtually all shipments of prescription drugs imported from (a foreign country) will run afoul of the Food Drug and Cosmetic Act "(FDCA)." This is due to their inability to comply with the FDCA regulations; the drug products from foreign countries must meet manufacturer-specific and product specific requirements, including:

- Manufacturing location
- Formulation
- Source and specifications of active ingredients
- Processing methods
- Manufacturing controls
- Container/closure systems
- Labeling

Out of desperation, many people continue to justify the practice by citing the "Personal Importation Policy" in the Food, Drug, & Cosmetic Act. This is the FDA policy that allows some patients and their doctors to import small quantities of *unapproved* drugs sold abroad for a patient's treatment of a serious condition for which effective treatment may not be available domestically. The FDA has made it abundantly clear that the policy is not intended to allow importation of foreign versions of drugs that are already *approved in the U.S.* Rather, the guidelines were created in order to allow critically ill patients to purchase experimental drugs as well as to permit prescription refills for travelers.

Many Americans are unaware that legislation was passed in 2000 entitled the Medicine Equity and Drug Safety Act (MEDS). MEDS actually allows reimportation if *the United States Secretary of the Department of Health and Human Services can determine that all the safety measures have been met.* Thus far, the three individuals who have held this office since 2000 (Donna Shalala, Tommy Thompson and now Mike Leavitt) have chosen not to pursue the controversial action of approving drug importation. According to past-Secretary Tommy G. Thompson, he "could not implement the act because it would sacrifice public safety by opening up the closed distribution system in the U.S."

The Pros and Cons of buying drugs from Canada

There are still <u>Pros</u> and <u>Cons</u>- advantages and disadvantages –in purchasing prescription drugs from Canada. Similar to the pros and cons involved in purchasing prescription drugs from U.S. Internet sites, they include:

Pros
1. <u>It's easy</u>. All a consumer needs to purchase drugs from a Canadian pharmacy is a credit card, a computer, and a phone line. It's also easy and quick to comparison-shop online.
2. <u>It may be cost-effective</u>: For U.S. brand name drugs, savings could be between 20-40%. Note: Anytime an advertisement claims up to an 80% discount, consider this a red flag. Usually there are just a few drugs with this deep of a discount from *legitimate* Canadian pharmacies.
3. <u>It affords privacy and anonymity</u>: Certainly, some consumers prefer privacy and anonymity for lifestyle drugs such as Viagra or

Propecia.
4. It may be convenient: It's often more convenient for those who live in rural areas or who have limited mobility to purchase prescription drugs online.

Cons
1. It's illegal: Although the U.S. government will probably never prosecute sick and elderly individuals, if they wanted to enforce the federal statutes, U.S. Customs laws and U.S. Postal laws, they could. Rather, it is more likely that the government will go after for-profit companies who lure in senior citizens and make a buck by breaking state/ federal laws.
2. It may be unsafe: Purchasing from an authentic, licensed Canadian website should technically be as safe as a U.S. Internet website but since the drugs are not FDA- approved there are never any guarantees. However, many experts believe that the regulations of Health Canada's Health Products and Food Branch are just as stringent and effective as the U.S. FDA, maybe even more so.
3. The quantities of doses often vary: Something that is very confusing for many Americans is that the *number* of pills in prescriptions filled by Canadian pharmacies is often different from the U.S. (e.g. 90-day supply in the U.S.; in Canada, it's a 100-day or bulk supply.) The 100-day supply ensures safety because the consumer is buying in bulk from an unopened bottle. This can be an inconvenience however, if the physician writes the prescription for just a 90-day supply. This would require the physician to make a call or re-write the prescription.
4. It might not actually be a reputable Canadian pharmacy. Unless you make a trip to a licensed Canadian pharmacy, or use an Internet site that has undergone a site review by a reputable company or government, you can never be sure the website represents a Canadian company. Everyone knows you can't believe everything you read on the Internet. A new FDA-commissioned study found that fewer than 2% of the thousands of websites claiming to sell Canadian prescription drugs were actually based in

Canada!

5. <u>Drugs should not be imported that are valued at more than $2,000.</u> Due to U.S. postal service requirements, the import of goods valued over $2,000 automatically requires a formal entry where the goods arrive in the U.S. If discovered by the U.S. Mail or U.S. Customs, the drugs can be held until the customer or designee can travel to the Customs mail branch and formerly enter the items.

6. <u>The FDA and or U.S Customs can confiscate the drugs at anytime.</u> Although they don't make a practice of it, the FDA and U.S. Customs have the authority to seize prescription drugs sent from Canada via mail bound for the U.S. or even from a tour bus crossing a land border. All of the packages containing prescription drugs are subject to search and seizure.

Actions for and against buying from Canada

As consumers, governments, and pharmaceutical companies argue the pros and cons of importation, *actions* for and against the practice continue. They include:

ACTIONS <u>FOR</u>

- 12 states and cities have implemented Canadian prescription importation programs and many more are considering it. Many cities and states are facing fiscal crises so it's easy to understand why they would seek ways to cut costs to the tune of hundreds of thousands of dollars. Take for example Springfield, Mass. During the first year of importation, the city saved $3 million by allowing some drugs to be purchased from Canada!

- Agencies that advocate for seniors such as AARP are continuing to support legislation to legalize the reimportation of drugs from Canada.

- Congressional representatives continue to draft Amendments to the new Medicare bill to include a provision for the legalization of importation of drugs from Canada

- Americans, exercising what they perceive as their right to free trade, continue to purchase prescription drugs from Internet sites at an increasing rate.

- Although it's illegal, U.S. government officials have stated that individuals who order prescription drugs from Canada or other foreign sources for their own use (up to 90 day quantities) will not being pursued or prosecuted.
- The Canadian International Pharmacy Association (CIPA) works on behalf of both the U.S. & Canada to promote buying prescription drugs from Canadian websites. However, CIPA *has* informed a number of state and local agencies in the U.S. that its 27-member mail order pharmacy association will <u>not</u> engage in *formal* commercial agreements. They continue to walk a very fine line, both politically and legally

ACTIONS <u>AGAINST</u>

- At least 4 of the Big Pharma companies have begun to fight back by **choking off** distribution of their prescription drugs to Canadian pharmacies that continue to send prescriptions to the U.S. According to Big Pharma, their contracts state that products are intended to be sold in the wholesaler's home market, i.e. Canada. If the pharmacies don't comply, pharmacies could lose significant revenue and create a possible shortage in Canada.
- The FDA continues to go after those that "aid and abet" the purchase of prescription drugs from Canada. For example, the FDA sent a warning letter to Expedite-Rx, the company assisting Montgomery employees in obtaining prescription drugs from Canada. Further action is pending. Also, the FDA has succeeded in prosecuting and closing two storefronts that acted as pharmacy intermediaries assisting consumers in obtaining drugs from Canada.
- 24 states have enacted laws to prevent the sale of prescriptions by other than a pharmacy licensed in that particular state. However, if the operations are *outside* of that particular state, (e.g. they don't have a storefront) then the operations are *not* under the jurisdiction of the State Pharmacy Boards and therefore they are unable to prosecute.
- Although the FDA is not going after seniors, the FDA does howev-

er, continue to implement their "Enforcement Actions Program" of both foreign and domestic websites by prosecuting those pharmacy websites that provide contaminated or adulterated drugs without a prescription or an examination from the patient's physician. As of April 2003, the FDA's enforcement actions included: 90 domestic Internet pharmacy investigations, 60 Internet pharmacy-related drug arrests, and 26 convictions.

Warnings

Prior to deciding to purchase prescription drugs from Canada or any foreign country, Americans should consider the following warnings:

1. Never buy prescriptions from a Canadian or any other Internet site that does not require a written prescription from the patient's health care professional. In addition to a written prescription, a history form should also be required.

2. Only purchase your prescription drugs only from a reputable Canadian pharmacy or Canadian pharmacy intermediary. The risks increase significantly when purchasing from foreign websites other than Canadian. IT'S JUST NOT WORTH IT. Be aware of what's known as "hiding under the maple leaf." This is the practice of web sites advertising themselves as Canadian or displaying the Canadian maple leaf flag when in fact they are not Canadian at all. For example, FDA investigators found three commonly prescribed drugs (Viagra, Lipitor, and Ambien) purchased from a website advertised as Canadian to be superpotent or subpotent. In actuality, the site was not a reputable Canadian website but instead operated from China with addresses in Miami and Dallas, with a toll-free number routed to Belize!

3. Be aware of the following types of risks that may be encountered with U.S. and foreign Internet websites:
   - Counterfeit or "fake" versions.
   - Adulterated versions, which are impure by added extraneous, improper, or inferior ingredients that alter the delivery or breakdown of the drug and its delivery.
   - Contaminated versions with potentially harmful substances,

such as bacteria.
- Drugs containing too little active, too much active ingredient, or none of the active ingredient at all.
- Drugs that are expired.
- Drugs that have been stored at the wrong temperature or under unsafe conditions.
- Drugs that are inappropriately packaged.

Note: Remember; take every precaution when purchasing prescription drugs from Canada.

Guidelines for purchasing prescription drugs from a Canadian land border

For those <u>still</u> considering hopping on a bus to purchase prescription drugs across a Canadian land border here are a few tips:
1. Take a valid prescription form as well as valid forms of identification (e.g. birth certificate/passport and driver's license.)
2. Be aware that a Canadian pharmacist needs to rewrite the prescription and that the name of the drug may be something entirely different in Canada. Always verify with the pharmacist that the prescription drug purchased is "therapeutically equivalent" to the one written on the U.S. prescription form.
3. Be advised that you can be stopped; the bus can be boarded by U.S. Customs, DEA and/or FDA agents. There is at least one publicized incident of this occurring.

Guidelines for purchasing prescription drugs from a Canadian Internet website

NOTE: THIS AUTHOR IS NOT CONDONING OR CONDEMNING THE PRACTICE OF BUYING PRESCRIPTION DRUGS IN CANADA. HOWEVER, AMERICANS SHOULD HAVE ACCESS TO THE MOST CURRENT AND ACCURATE INFORMATION REGARDING THIS ISSUE.

CHECK THE AUTHOR'S WEBSITE AT <u>WWW.PRESCRIPTIONPATHWAY.COM</u> FOR UPDATES ON LEGAL ISSUES REGARDING PURCHASING PRE-SCRIPTION DRUGS IN CANADA.

If readers are <u>still</u> considering purchasing from a Canadian *Internet web-site* after knowing that it is illegal, then they should follow *all* of the five tips below:

1. <u>For every prescription(s), consult with your health care profes-sionals to determine if you need to take any special steps for fill-ing your prescription in Canada.</u> Ask your physicians if you can purchase your prescription from a reputable Canadian Internet website after the first 30 days of treatment. NEVER BUY FROM CANADA UNTIL YOU HAVE BEEN ON A PRESCRIPTION DRUG FOR MORE THAN 30 DAYS. Ask if you can have drug samples for the first 30 days and then a written prescription for 100 tablets after that. If drug samples are unavailable, ask for two prescriptions, one for 30 days, and one for 100 tablets. This gives you time to see if you can tolerate the medication and to receive one-on-one prescribing instructions from your health care profes-sional and/or pharmacist. You can also read about the drug using the package insert or a reputable drug guide. In addition, the new medication needs to be added to your list of chronic medications at your local pharmacy, which ensures there won't be any food-drug or drug-drug interactions. Remember: your own primary care provider knows more about your health and what prescrip-tions you should be taking than any other person. Remember that you will never have a satisfactory *physician-patient* relationship with a website.

2. <u>Find a resource that can identify credible Canadian Internet web-sites.</u> One such source is <u>www.pharmacychecker.com</u>. This website checks to see if online pharmacies meet certain criteria. (The cri-teria are very similar to the FDA recommendations listed in Chapter 12.) Each pharmacy and pharmacy intermediary is given a "1-5 star rating." This author recommends using only 5-star rated companies, but each consumer ultimately makes his or her own personal choice. PharmacyChecker.com membership is $19.95 per year, but the cost can be well worth it. Consumers can

also check prescription prices on this web site at no charge.

3. <u>Check the table of 30 medications listed in this chapter to determine if savings will be substantial enough to buy the drugs from Canada.</u> Then use the price comparison tool in APPENDIX **A** and complete the form found in APPENDIX **D** to ensure that there will enough of a savings to outweigh any associated risks.

4. <u>Follow the instructions of the online pharmacy by completing all the forms truthfully</u>. Forms include, but are not limited to: a history questionnaire and a consent form.

5. <u>Review the Prescription Pathways in Chapter 16</u>. Then determine if your personal "prescription pathway" might lead to purchasing

---

It Could Happen to You

John Smith is a 29-year-old film producer who regretfully lacks a steady income. Like many working poor, he has been uninsured for ten years. With money being tight, he decided to purchase his prescription drugs at a Canadian Internet site (Zoloft 50 mg, once daily for 90 days). After asking for his physician's approval, John obtained a prescription for *100 mg.* tablets (90 of them) so that the pills could be split to provide 50 mg. doses for *180 days* of therapy. Upon reviewing several Canadian websites on www.pharmacychecker.com, he decided to purchase from www.canadameds.com. The cost quoted at that time was $125. If he were to purchase the same amount and dose of Zoloft at *Costco*, the cost would have been $210. John's written prescription was faxed in to Canadameds.com and he began the 14-21 day waiting period for his shipment to arrive. About two weeks later, he received a call from an employee of Canadameds.com and was informed that they didn't have the *100 mg.* in stock and would he like to purchase the 50 mg. instead? Since he had already waited 2 weeks and he knew it would be another 1-2 weeks delay, he agreed. The cost for the Zoloft *50 mg.* for 100 tablets was $123.45 or $1.23 per pill. *Therefore, as it turned out, it would have been the <u>same</u> price to purchase the 100-mg. tabs from Costco for $210 because he would have had twice the number of doses once he split the tablets! In addition, he wouldn't*

> *have had to worry about legal issues and he wouldn't have had to wait for 14-21 days for therapy for begin.*
>
> **Outcome:**   **$1.23 per dose from Canadameds.com (50 mg.)**
> **Could have been:**   **$1.23 per dose from Costco- (100 mg.- split)**
>
> He also received 100 tablets instead of 90, which has been an issue with the FDA (known as illegal prescribing due to the fact that the number prescribed exceeded the number written on the prescription.) However, receiving the 100-tablet bottle assured a bulk order, with the bottle still *sealed by the manufacturer*. There is less of a chance of tampering or counterfeiting when receiving the original tablets in bulk.

from Canadian Internet sites or if there is a better option for you. In the long run, your best choice for safety and convenience will always be purchases from the U.S.

Consumer Information

For more information on U.S. prescription drug laws regarding importation, please refer to:

1. U.S. Food and Drug Administration: www.fda.gov
2. U.S. Customs Office: www.customs.gov
3. U.S. trade office: www.ustr.gov

See also the FDA's article: "Buying Medicines and Medical Products Online" at *www.fda.gov*.

Conclusion

The tug of war concerning reimportation from Canada is far from over. With at least two drug importation bills being considered by Congress in 2005, it's difficult to read the crystal ball and know what the future will bring. One thing for sure is that there are special interest groups on both sides of the issue that will continue to fight for their cause. And caught in the middle are seniors, disabled and uninsured Americans. Many state officials and citizen groups have asked that, at the very least, a waiver be provided to individual Americans who are buying prescription drugs from Canada or Europe for just themselves or their families. This would allow them to purchase the drugs without fear of reprisal or incarceration. To date, there are no measures to protect these individuals.

In November 2004, the Canadian Health Minister was quoted at a speech at Harvard Medical School as saying: "It is difficult to conceive how a country such as Canada which is one-tenth the size of the U.S. could meet the prescription drug needs of America's 280 million citizens." He estimates that Internet pharmacy sales of prescription drugs to the U.S. have reached a plateau at $700 million annually. He has also made it clear that he does not want to be the drugstore for the U.S. In fact, Canadian Health Minister Ujjal Dosanjh is planning on implementing a ban on bulk imports (but fortunately, not a ban on Canadian online pharmacy sales to individuals). In the meantime, Canadian pharmacy intermediaries will probably continue to create agreements with other countries, especially Europe. It has been reported that approximately *three quarters* of the legitimate Canadian pharmacies have developed agreements with other countries such as Israel, the U.K., Australia, and New Zealand in order to keep up with U.S. demand. In addition, the *number* of legitimate Canadian Internet pharmacies has decreased by half since all the importation difficulties escalated in 2005.

In conclusion, consumers and advocacy groups need to continue to bring issues such as reimportation and the high cost of prescription drugs front and center, whether they buy from Canada or not. Keeping the reimportation controversy politically charged will hopefully bring about a positive impact on drug prices in the future.

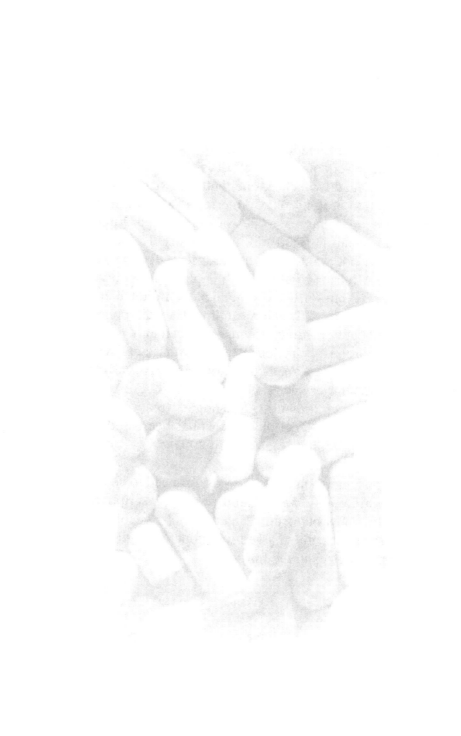

PART IV: BUYING PRESCRIPTION DRUGS IN EUROPE

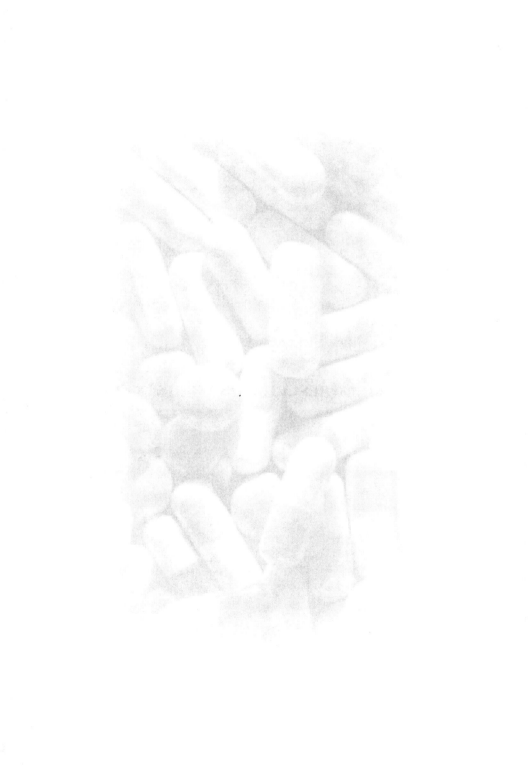

Chapter 14

If not Canada, try Europe

Introduction

Due to the many regulations and political ploys recently restricting the cross-border trade for prescription drugs from Canada, certain countries in Europe are becoming increasingly popular locations for Americans who want to buy prescription drugs via the Internet. In fact, the majority of Canadian pharmacies/pharmacy intermediaries have begun to negotiate contracts in Europe to provide an adequate supply of brand name prescription drugs to their American customers. Many of the companies have had to create the networks under the cloak of secrecy so that the same thing that happened in Canada with Big Pharma choking off the drug supply doesn't happen in Europe as well.

It's no wonder that pharmacies believe secrecy is vital. Many trade experts in Europe worry that this increase in parallel trade (See Chapter 13) will ignite a bidding war between Canadian, European and American consumers for the most popular drugs-thereby forcing global drug prices higher, not lower.[1] Drugmakers are concerned that a surge in imports from Europe may undermine their control over global distribution of their products. The drug companies sell *seven* times more drugs by value in the 25-nation European Union than they do in Canada, so Europe has far bigger supplies of inexpensive medicines that could be exported for U.S. customers.[2] Big Pharma, of course, is already considering tightening controls on European supplies to stop the flow of low-cost products into the U.S. In fact, Richard Freudenberg, secretary general of the British Association of European Pharmaceutical Distributors, says Pfizer is already trying to restrict Europe's cross-border trade.

Many are also concerned that the drugs through parallel trading in the EU might not be safe. The prescription drugs often change hands as many as 20 times! And as discussed in Chapter 3, the more times that the drugs change hands, the higher the potential for counterfeiting. Yet, Europeans don't seem to be too worried, based on historical information. This however, was *before* Americans starting buying prescription drugs from the EU against the advice and regulations of the FDA.

Cost Savings are substantial

As with Canada, the reason for this importation from Europe is simple: money! As reported by reliable sources, for consumers accustomed to paying U.S. prices, a European supplier can save them *big* money: For example, a three-month supply of 500- milligram tablets of Glucophage diabetes medicine, which sells for $65.52 in the U.S., can be bought in Ireland for the equivalent of $16.90, a _74%_ savings. A three-month supply of Nexium ulcer medication, selling for $751 in the U.S., costs less than half that, or about $342, in the U.K.

In 2004, the European Union's (EU) total drug sales were approximately $92 billion compared with over $200 billion for the U.S. The U.S. has only 2/3 of the population of the EU but accounts for more than double the sales revenue for Big Pharma.[3]

Already, Americans have problems importing from Europe

Customers of Governor of Illinois Rod Blagojevich's I-SaveRX program (importation program for Illinois state residents) are already having problems receiving their prescription drugs ordered from the U.K via their website. In fact, since January 2005, 54 customers of I-Save Rx have already reported that the FDA has seized shipments of their medications, including Pfizer's Lipitor cholesterol drug sent from the U.K. As with Canada, the importation is breaking U.S. laws, not U.K. laws, as it *is legal* for the U.K. pharmacies to export the drugs from the U.K., as long as a U.K.-registered physician signs the prescriptions.

Governor Blagojevich has now stated that Australia and New Zealand will be added to the I-SaveRX program later this year. Australia will fill most prescription drugs and New Zealand will fill prescription drugs that are available over-the-counter in their country. Australian prices are approximately 51% less than in the U.S.[4]

Conclusion

What this author calls the "Importation Wars" has already begun in Europe. So what do Americans do? They reach out to other countries such as New Zealand, Israel, and Australia. Even India has become a popular importation location. Notice that China is not mentioned. CHINA IS BAD NEWS. Currently 90% of the drugs in China are counterfeit.

Many readers will probably find the "Importation Wars" silly, confusing, frustrating, or maybe just downright disgusting. The author can identify with all these sentiments. **The entire system is broken** if it requires such drastic measures from both sides. There are no easy answers, but many believe the Importation Wars would never have gotten this bad in the first place if brand name drugs had been more affordable to uninsured Americans.

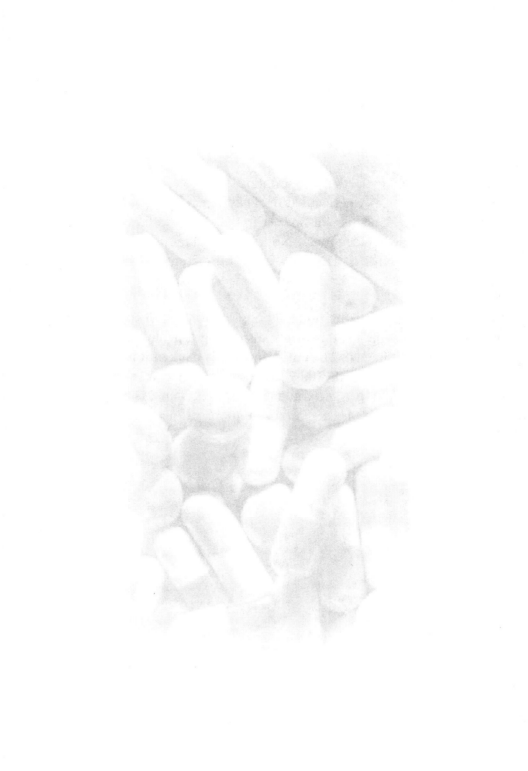

PART V   BUYING PRESCRIPTION DRUGS IN MEXICO

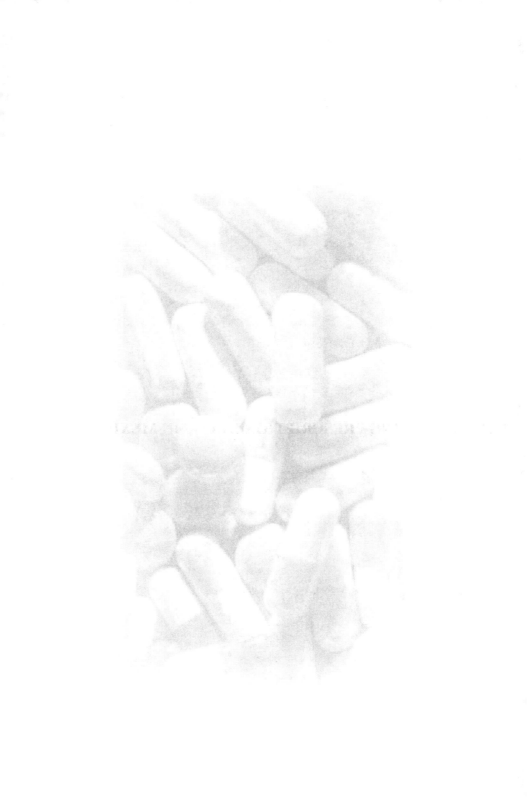

Chapter 15

ADIOS MEXICO!

> **TIP: JUST SAY NO to buying prescription drugs in Mexico. Check out Prescription Pathways in Chapter 16 for better, safer alternatives.**

Introduction

Americans who have grown up in a state bordering Mexico (i.e. Arizona, Texas, and California) have long been known to drive across the border to purchase merchandise. It's a fun way to spend a Saturday afternoon; pack up the car and the kids and head to the border for some shopping. The hot items in the 1970s and 1980s were piñatas, leather apparel, pottery, glassware, furniture, baskets, rugs, and jewelry.

But times have changed. Over the past few years, as prescription drug costs have continued to skyrocket in the U.S., Mexican border towns are now a hotbed for what this author calls: "The legal drug trade" or "the other drug problem." In other words, Americans (and others) are purchasing prescription drugs from Mexican pharmacies and bringing them across the land border into the United States. This has become a major source of income and tourist trade for border towns in Mexico. Currently, it's estimated that $800 million in prescription drugs are being exported from Mexico!

Like Canada, Americans can purchase prescription drugs from Mexico, either by actually traveling to Mexico or by purchasing them via the Internet.

LIKE CANADA, PURCHASING PRESCRIPTION DRUGS FROM MEXICO (OTHER THAN IN AN EMERGENCY SITUATION) AND IMPORTING THEM INTO THE U.S. IS ILLEGAL. MORE IMPOR-

TANTLY, IT IS UNSAFE!
A common practice- why do Americans do it?

According to the Federal Consumer Information Center, 15-16 million U.S. Citizens visit Mexico each year. It's estimated that 40% of these consumers will return with prescription drugs. While on the surface, this situation may *seem* identical to Canada; there are additional safety concerns when purchasing any drugs from Mexico.

The pros and cons of buying prescription drugs in Mexico

Pros
1. It's Easy. U.S. citizens visiting Mexico in the "border zone" for no more than 72 hours are not required to have a passport or permit to walk or drive across the border. Plus, just a few blocks from the International borders are dozens of Farmacias (pharmacies). In fact, it's so easy to buy prescription drugs in Mexico border towns that it's similar to buying candy in a grocery store. Often, a shopper just has to request a drug and it is brought to the counter, without any patient counseling, proof of a prescription form, etc.

2. It may save money. Generics sold in Mexico are very inexpensive. However, surprisingly, when buying a *brand name* drug in Mexico, the price is similar to the U.S., unless of course an individual wants to "haggle" or barter. For example, in 2003 at a Nogales, Mexico farmacia, Zocor 10mg-30-day supply, cost $71.16. This was similar to U.S. prices at the time. However, purchasing a *generic* version of Lipitor 20 mg cost just $105.00 for *100*. This is a deep, deep discount from U.S. prices. (Note: there is *no FDA-approved* generic version of Lipitor).

Cons
1. It's illegal. As with Canada, **hypothetically** speaking, it should be possible to legally purchase a 30-day supply of a prescription drug from Mexico *for personal use,* if the consumer has a valid prescription. As with other foreign countries, both a U.S. pre-

scription form and a local-(Mexico) prescription form are required. (Note: Most Mexican farmacias will provide referrals to a physician right down the street who will write a prescription for a small fee, *without* completing a health questionnaire or taking a history and/or physical.) In addition, in order for the prescription drug purchase to be legal, it must be FDA-approved and be made by an FDA-approved manufacturer that has the approval to manufacture that *specific* drug. It must also meet U.S. requirements for FDA- approved labeling, packaging, and manufacturing, which differs greatly from the requirements in Mexico. Therefore, **practically** speaking, it's virtually impossible that a drug purchased from Mexico (or Canada or Europe!) will meet all these requirements as mentioned and will therefore be considered illegal in accordance with FDA and U.S. Customs.

Legally, the negative consequences of buying prescription drugs in Mexico can be minor or they can be catastrophic! Consider an elderly gentleman arrested in Nogales, Mexico in 2004 for buying 270 tablets of Valium for his wife using his wife's U.S. prescription form. At the same time this individual was in a Nogales JAIL, there were 11 other Arizonans being held as part of a crackdown of people buying tranquilizers and painkillers without a legitimate prescription. After almost 8 weeks, this unassuming Arizona senior citizen was finally released. The moral of the story: Although most of the problems in this particular instance were likely due to the fact that he purchased a *controlled* substance (Valium), many would agree that perhaps *it's best not to purchase prescription drugs in Mexico.*

2. It's unsafe.

At the present time, experts agree that purchasing prescription drugs from Mexican pharmacies or from websites advertised as Mexican pharmacies is infinitely more risky than purchasing them in the U.S. or even Canada. Reasons for safety concerns include:

a. Language barriers: Unless the consumer is bi-lingual, there may be language barriers to overcome in the buying process. Prescription drug prescribing and purchasing is a very individ ualized process and many nuances can be lost in translation.

b. Most Mexican pharmacies are not licensed.

c. Most experts do not believe that the drug system is as well regulated in Mexico as in the U.S., Canada, Australia, or Europe.

Specific safety hazards include:

a. Counterfeit drugs- Counterfeit drugs have already been dis cussed in length, but its worth mentioning that **counter- feit** drugs shipped from a Mexican pharmacy website have indeed been identified more than once.

b. Contaminated Drugs- It happens. Last year, two children were killed from contaminated penicillin purchased in Mexico.

c. Subpotent or superpotent drugs- Many of the prescription and over-the-counter drugs for sale from Mexico that have been seized during raids conducted by U.S. Customs and the FDA have been found to be *subpotent*, meaning they contain less active ingredient than is stated on the prescription box or label. For example, some antibiotics sold in Mexico that were ana lyzed by U.S. labs contained only 1/10 of the active ingredient listed. The FDA also identified generic Evista, counterfeit Lipitor, and Viagra products that contained no active ingredi ent at all. If the drug purchased is a version of a lifestyle drug like Viagra or Retin-A, subpotency is relatively harmless. However, if a life saving heart medication or blood pressure medication is subpotent, it can be *fatal*. Drugs may also be *superpotent* (contain too much active ingredient), but this is less likely.

d. Expired drugs- Consumers may be purchasing expired drugs without their knowledge. Expired drugs run the risk of being subpotent as well.

e. Fillers- Drugs manufactured and/or purchased from Mexico may have different volumes or types of fillers (inactive ingre dients). This can affect the rate of the drug's distribution and therefore the drug will not be bioequivalent. Toxic substances such as chromium and lead have been found as added fillers in medications imported from Mexico.

f. Similares- Latin American countries have a different class of drugs known as similares. They are copycat products that are sold legally but have not been tested for bioequivalency or quality. Although there are new bioequivalency requirements for true generics, the similares are a "gray area." A consumer buying a "generic" from a farmacia wouldn't be able to tell the difference.

It Could Happen to You

"Field Trip to Mexico":

As"field research" for the book, the author took a field trip to Nogales, Mexico in June 2003. After speaking with a customs agent at the international border crossing and informing him that she would be purchasing prescription drugs, she was told that she could bring back 50 pills without a prescription. As she walked up and down the main street that has turned into a "pharmacy strip," she spoke to several Mexican pharmacists and assistants. Everyone was very helpful and accommodating.

The most remarkable experience happened when she came across a "hawker" standing in front of a farmacia, yelling the words: "We have Lipitor, Prozac, *and Valium!* Holding onto a camera and a note pad, she asked him: "Do you really have Valium, how much is it"? At that point the hawker asked if she was a cop and then walked away. (Reminder: Valium is a controlled substance and has addictive properties.) Everyone known to be arrested crossing the border in Nogales this year has been in possession of one or more controlled substances so this is a very dangerous practice for Americans.

The author also tried to slip up an employee in a farmacia by asking her for medical advice. The author asked the assistant if she could take Lopid and Zocor together. The assistant acted appropriately and told her to check with her doctor (Note: taking Zocor with Lopid can potentially lead to severe drug interactions.)

Lastly, the author walked into a farmacia and asked for first one drug, then changed her mind and asked for a different drug then changed it back again. She was never asked for a prescription for any of her purchases (and they were more than a 50 day supply). At the border, she declared her drug purchases, but was never asked to produce them (they were in a plastic bag).

Picture from the field trip to Nogales, Mexico-A Street the author calls "Farmacia Row":

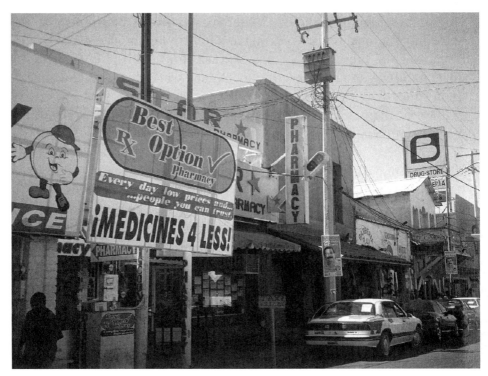

Conclusion

When evaluating the "value" of shopping for prescription drugs from Mexican pharmacies, whether in a border town or via the Internet, individuals need to weigh the cost benefits vs. the *legal and safety* risks. Since purchasing certain subpotent or fake drugs could cost a patient his or her life, one has to consider if it is really worth it. One might make the argument that certain lifestyle drugs (such as Retin-A or Propecia) might be acceptable *in a healthy individual with no underlying diseases.* The reason would be that if the lifestyle drug contained little or no active ingredient, there would be minimal risks. However, the drug(s) could still contain other harmful (or deadly) active or inactive ingredients or fillers.

If readers, after weighing all the risks, still believe they absolutely must still purchase drugs from Mexico (against the advice of informed experts), then the following <u>8</u> tips for purchasing prescription drugs should be followed.

1. Consult with your personal physician regarding whether it would be *appropriate* to purchase your specific medications in Mexico. *If* the physician says yes, carry an up-to-date copy of the U.S. prescription.
2. Obtain a prescription from a Mexican doctor. (Most Mexican pharmacies will help you.)
3. Keep a copy of all prescription forms.
4. Only buy medications prescribed for your own use.
5. DO NOT BUY CONTROLLED SUBSTANCES.
6. Obtain a receipt from the Mexican pharmacy.
7. Be sure to get the correct medication and dosage.
8. Do not buy more than a one month supply.
9. Declare all purchased medications when re-entering the United States.
10. If any reactions to medications occur, call your physician immediately![1]

The *author's recommendation* is to use the "Prescription Pathways" outlined in this book to find safe, yet cost-effective, alternatives to buying prescription drugs from Mexico.

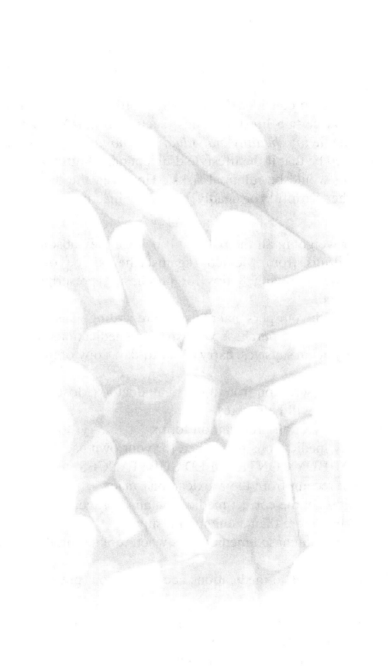

PART VI   PRESCRIPTION PATHWAYS

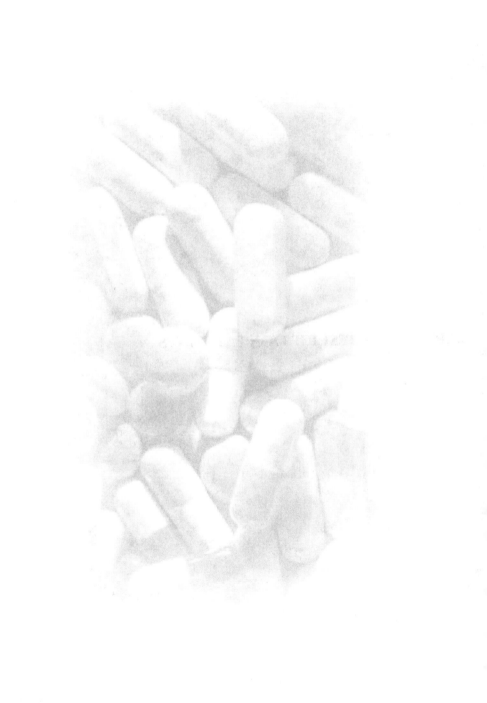

Chapter 16
Find *Your* Prescription Pathway

Every reader should find his or her own "Prescription Pathway." The personalized pathway will aid the reader in comparison-shopping and finding the best value. Three are listed in this chapter. More can be found on www.prescriptionpathway.com.

Pathway A: General Prescription Pathway for all Medicare individuals

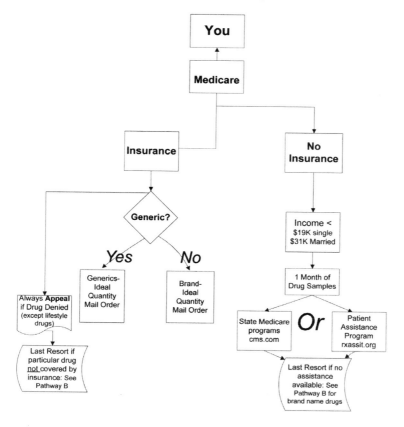

Note: This Medicare Pathway will be updated on the author's website (www.prescriptionpathway.com) after January 2006.

Pathway B: Prescription Pathway for *Brand Name* Drugs

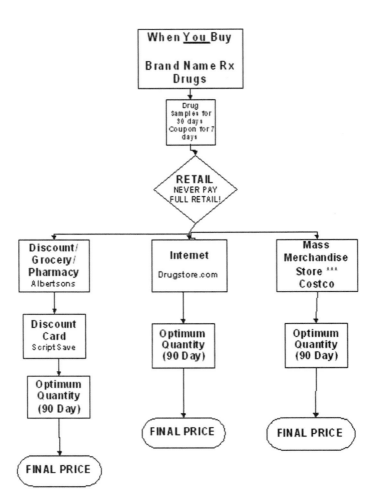

***Note: Costco is the preferred choice for both safety & convenience. After that, www.drugstore.com is 1st choice based on price and then Albertsons/Osco with a ScriptSave card is a choice based on convenience.

Pathway C: Example- Lipitor 20 mg.

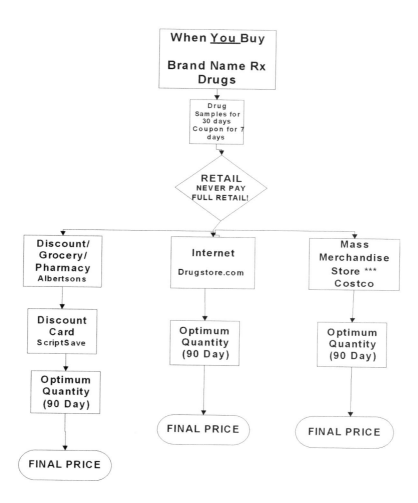

Note: Prices are for comparison purposes only and subject to change. Prices may also vary by region.

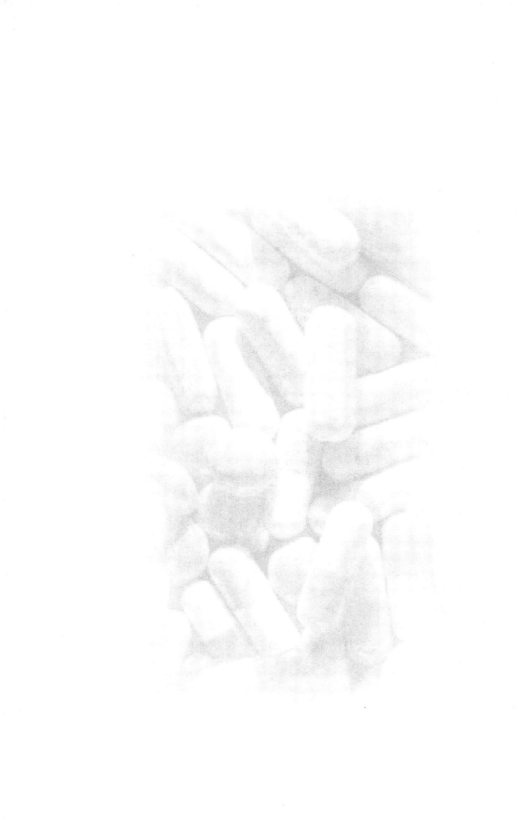

Chapter 17

Rx Tune-up

TIP: As part of an Rx Tune-up, use the Prescription Pathways to find discounts. Check the website: www.prescriptionpathway.com for updates.

Equipped with all the information in the previous chapters, readers may now want to perform an "Rx Tune-up." This is a review and revamp of all prescription drug records and purchases.

Consumers routinely take their cars in for a tune-up and maintenance, but yet they neglect their health. Updating drug therapy information can be a vital part of a routine "tune up" or health "face-lift." Comparison-shopping can be done in conjunction with the tune-up.

Steps to your Rx Tune-up include:

1. **Clean out your medicine cabinet:** Go through your medicine cabinet and any kitchen/bathroom cabinets that have prescription drugs, OTC medications, and dietary/herbal supplements and look for bottles or cartons that have expired and/or that you are no longer using. Dispose of all of these medications and supplements. This is the first step to your Rx Tune-up.

2. **Schedule an appointment with your healthcare practitioner**: Readers should schedule an appointment with their primary care practitioner if one is not already scheduled in the near future. At that time an "Rx Tune-up" can be done along with an updated physical or mini-physical.

3. **Complete a new medication list**: An up-to-date medication is vital _prior_ to prescription drug comparison-shopping. It is recommended that you use the checkbook medication record included in APPENDIX C or another approved medication record provided by your physician. You can also use the medication record recommended by the National Council on Patient Information and

Education (NCPIE) - see www.talkaboutrx.org. Be sure to include all OTC medications as well as dietary and herbal supplements on the medication record.

4. **Ask for new prescriptions at your doctor's appointment:** With a new medication record, readers can then ask for new prescription forms at the next doctor's appointment. If the prescription forms are for chronic medications, ask for a prescription for a 90-100 day supply. (Be advised that if the desire is to order from a *reputable* Canadian website, the prescription will probably need to be for 100 tablets/capsules. This is the size of a bulk bottle that is sealed and therefore safer). ALWAYS MAKE A COPY OF THE ORIGINAL PRESCRIPTION FORMS FOR YOUR RECORDS.

5. **Review the Prescription Pathways in this book and find your own unique path**: Determine the appropriate pathway-Medicare or Non-Medicare, low income or moderate income, insurance or no insurance, etc. THIS IS THE STEP WHERE THE COMPARISON SHOPPING HAPPENS. If necessary, check websites for prices, or call the local pharmacies. Use the price comparison tool in APPENDIX A. Ask your physician or pharmacist if you have questions.

6. **Pick a pharmacy "Home":** Make a decision on whether you want to make purchases from a brick-and-mortar pharmacy, an Internet pharmacy, or a pharmacy/pharmacy intermediary that has both. *Then pick one pharmacy to be your "home."* If there is a discount card for which you need to enroll in order to take advantage of this new "home," make sure you officially enroll *prior* to making your prescription drug purchases.

7. **Check www.prescriptionpathway.com:** Review the author's website for any updates on counterfeit drugs or other newsworthy items that might affect your purchases. The website will have additional cost saving tips and prescription pathways.

8. **Re-evaluate your pharmacy profile every 6 months**: Once a tune-up has been completed, be sure to re-evaluate your drug product purchases as well as your prescription pathway every 6 months for a "mini-tune-up."

<u>Happy Shopping!</u>

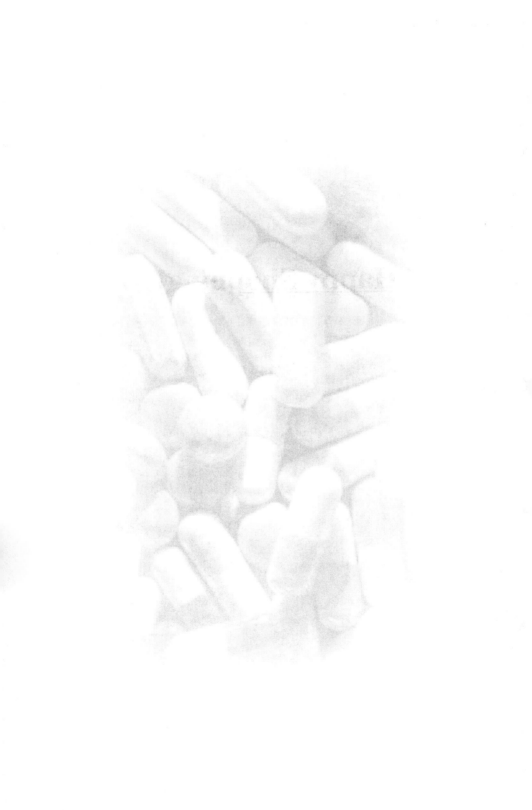

Chapter 18

A Look to the Future

The next few years will be exciting times in the world of pharmaceuticals and biotechnology. As costs continue to increase, so will the wonderful opportunities for new, improved drug therapy. This chapter is just a brief look at a few of the highlights ahead.

One step forward, two steps back

Just when it appears the U.S. is taking a step forward, certain practices and policies put us two steps behind. Listed below are just a few examples to contemplate:

1. Medicare-Many politicians considered Medicare a triumph for the elderly and disabled, but many *Medicare recipients* feel differently. Many Americans hoped that a new Medicare prescription drug benefit would allow the elderly to have a total comprehensive package that encompassed all medically necessary prescription drug purchases. This didn't happen. With the new law, there are copays, deductibles, doughnut hole, loopholes, and formularies. The first testament to what should have been a *positive* feature of the new law was the Medicare-approved Prescription Drug Discount Card Program. This program, however, was disappointing. The jury is still out on the "full" Medicare prescription drug benefit. Policy makers and advocates will be watching this one closely.

2. Once-a-month medications- Drug companies are looking at developing monthly medications (pills or even injectables) that would be taken only once every 1, 3 or 6 months. In fact, in March 2005, the FDA approved the first once-a-month pill, Boniva, to treats osteoporosis. As a pharmacy technician, the author sees this is a

great step forward in patient compliance. What is disturbing, however, is that the drug companies intend to charge the same amount as they would with a regular bottle of pills, even though the monthly pills cost less to manufacturer! Cost savings are indeed possible with advances in pharmacotherapy, but rarely are the savings passed onto the consumer.

3. Clinical trials conducted in other countries- This is another example of a cost savings strategy employed by Big Pharma. In fact, as discussed in Chapter 5, many drug companies have already started conducting clinical trials in third world countries such as India in order to cut costs. So far, these savings have not been passed on to the consumer.

4. New drug-safety monitoring office: Due to the media and litigation surrounding VIOXX and other COX-2 inhibitors, the FDA is planning on creating an office or division in the FDA that steps up the monitoring of drugs in the *post*-market phase. Money has been set aside to make this a reality. But there is a trade off. As the FDA steps forward on this front, they have announced that there will be *less* money to complete FDA inspections on manufacturing facilities, both here in the U.S. and abroad. Normally, there are approximately 3,500 inspections a year and many believe more are needed, not less. But in order to pay for "safety" in one area, they will be sacrificing safety in another.

5. Biotech- Biotechnology will continue to take the forefront in drug development in the next decade. What remains to be seen is *who* will be paying the tab. As discussed in Chapter 2, some of these drugs, i.e. chemotherapy drugs, may cost $40,000 per patient- this is more than double the cost of the drugs available *prior* to biotech. Many people believe in the phrase coined by Dr Stephen Schondelmeyer from the University Of Minnesota School Of Pharmacy: "A drug that is not affordable is neither safe nor effective."

6. Comparison-shopping within the same therapeutic class: In addition to comparison-shopping for a better price on the *same* drug, some government and health care officials are advocating buying a less expensive drug in the *same drug class*. To begin, compar-

isons are being made for prescription and non-prescription drugs for drug classes that treat cholesterol, pain, and heartburn. For example, Lipitor is compared to other statins using criteria such as average expected LDL reduction, proven reduction of the risk of heart attacks, proven mortality reduction and lastly, price. Consumers Union, a nonprofit publisher of Consumer Reports, also has a website that compares and contrasts prescription drugs *in the same drug class,* according to safety and effectiveness and combines evidence-based research with national-level data on drug prices. The www.medicare.gov website also includes evidence-based information on some therapeutic classes. Most of the websites are using information from the Drug Effectiveness Review Project (DERP), a 12-state initiative (See Chapter 3). Comparing drugs for efficacy *and cost* by independent parties are the wave of the future.

7. *Behind*-the-Counter: This is a new alternative for a class of drugs in between prescription and non-prescription drugs. BTC designation is one way to prevent the abuse of common OTC drugs as well as a way to control the use and education of drugs such as an OTC cholesterol drug and the infamous "Plan B" drug, which is a prescription emergency contraception pill. Laws governing the FDA do not recognize a BTC class, and new federal legislation would be required to establish such a system. Nevertheless, some states are adopting laws that would at least restrict sales of popular OTC drugs used to make illegal methamphetamines. Oklahoma, who was once one of the top states in the illegal manufacture of methamphetamines, has been able to attack the problem successfully by keeping the OTCs behind the pharmacy counter and by restricting the number of boxes sold.

8. Listing prescription prices: There are many ways to make prescription costs more transparent. Some of the ideas being implemented or reviewed include: 1) Print on the receipt and/or pill bottle the true cost of the prescription drug as well as what a consumer pays, 2) Provide price lists at the pharmacy and 3) Require PBMs to make their price negotiations available to consumers. Many states are looking at initiatives such as these to provide cost

savings to local and state governments. The purpose of this transparency would be to actually decrease drug prices, however, many believe this could backfire and cause the opposite to happen. Although the strategies that will ultimately be implemented in the future may vary, transparency and education are sure to play a major part.

Individualization

One of the most exciting advances in drug therapy is known as "pharmacogenomics." This science develops gene tests to help tailor prescriptions to each patient's DNA. For decades, scientists have known that individual patients will react differently to drugs, based on many factors including how fast a drug is metabolized. This can affect whether a drug can climb to toxic levels in some patients or conversely, clear the patient's bloodstream before it can have the desired effect. There is now a test that will allow physicians to determine the level of certain enzymes in the body that can have these effects; the AmpliChip CYP450 was cleared by the FDA in December 2004 and was scheduled to be available by June 2005. Perhaps physicians will now believe their patients when they tell them that a drug has made them really sick or has had no effect, rather than assuming it "was all in their head". This author believes this "individualization" of drug therapy will be one of our greatest developments in the next decade.

Globalization & Importation

Globalization and importation are buzzwords that Americans will continue to hear more about in relation to prescription drugs. Regarding globalization, drug companies will continue to merge and will also continue to create manufacturing plants around the globe. They will continue to outsource certain business practices and the world will continue to become smaller place.

Importation, although very controversial, will continue to be a hot topic. It's very possible that by the end of 2005 Congress will pass some type of reimportation legislation. However, the author believes that there will be very little "teeth" in the legislation because the drug industry lobby is still too powerful. Nonetheless, consumers and advocacy groups will continue to make reimportation an issue unless some kinds of price controls are implemented to curtail the high cost of brand name prescription drugs.

Last, but not least

The author experienced a lot of raised eyebrows in the healthcare community when first revealing two years ago that she was writing a book on comparison-shopping and buying prescription drugs in the U.S., Canada, and other countries. However, since then, nearly *all-political,* and public leaders have come forward and suggested that Americans shop around and compare prices. This trend is now here to stay, as consumers feel more empowered and gain a desire to participate in their own health care. Consumers may not always be able to control the prescription drug prices that are set, but they *can* control which retail outlet they use. Nevertheless, comparison-shopping should never be done without sufficient knowledge and a set of "tools" with which to aid in making informed choices. Hopefully this book will be a step in the right direction.

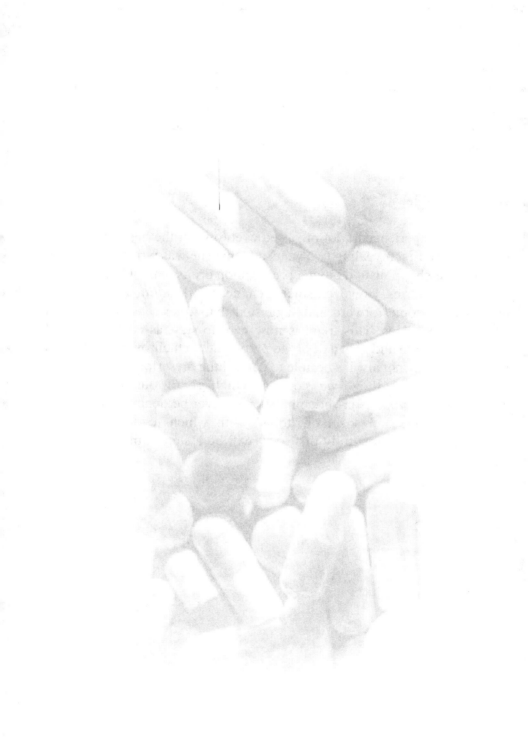

APPENDIX A

APPENDIX A
Prices for the Top 100 Drugs Prescribed

The following price comparisons are designed to assist readers in making purchasing decisions for prescription drugs. The chart emphasizes the price ranges between retailers in the U.S., Canada and on the Internet in *June 2005*. (**The lowest price is typed in bold**). When possible, prices were obtained for a 90-100 day quantity. However, quantities vary and therefore, a price per dose was also calculated. When there is a generic equivalent available for the brand drug, the generic name is in parentheses and then also listed under its generic name (alphabetically). Note: Shipping charges are not included. (All drugs are tablets unless otherwise noted) Note: N/A = Not Available

Drug Name & Dose Brand-UPPER CASE Generics- lower case	Mass Merchant Selling Price	Mass Merchant Unit Cost	Drug Chain Selling Price	Drug Chain Unit Cost	U.S. Internet pharmacy Selling Price	U.S. Internet pharmacy Unit Cost	Canadian Internet pharmacy Selling price	Canada Internet pharmacy Unit Cost
Albuterol 90mcg inhaler 17gm (3)	14.58	**4.86**	44.29	11.76	35.99	12.00	N/A	N/A
ALLEGRA 180MG	221.67	2.22	191.97	2.22	191.97	2.13	45.00	**1.50**
Allopurinol 300mg	18.19	.18	3391	.18	15.99	**.16**	N/A	N/A
AMBIEN 10mg	296.57	2.97	269.09	2.99	233.97	**2.60**	N/A	N/A
Amitriptyline HCL 25mg	14.37	.14	27.69	.15	10.99	**.12**	26.71	.27
Atenolol 30mg	7.99	**.08**	11.89	.20	10.99	.12	41.42	.41
AVANDIA 4mg	269.99	2.70	252.49	2.81	238.95	2.66	271.04	**2.61**
Bupropion hcl 100mg	34.39	**.34**	80.99	.80	69.99	1.17	N/A	N/A
Captopril 25mg	21.07	.21	18.99	.19	14.99	**.15**	52.78	.52
CARDIZEM CD 240MG CAP SA (diltiazem hcl	213.57	**2.14**	215.99	2.4	N/A	N/A	N/A	N/A
CARDURA 4MG (Doxazosin mesylate)	121.49	**1.21**	81.99	1.36	N/A	N/A	131.02	1.31
CELEBREX 100MG	170.37	1.70	119.99	2.00	95.99	1.60	96.80	**.97**
CELEBREX 200MG	326.95	3.27	175.99	2.93	227.97	2.53	174.67	**1.75**
CELEXA 20 MG	243.59	2.44	216.39	2.40	194.97	2.17	50.27	**1.68**
CIALIS 10 MG	922.27	9.22	335.89	11.20	269.97	**9.00**	N/A	N/A
CLARINEX 5MG	216.77	2.17	196.99	2.19	188.97	2.10	113.96	**1.13**
CRESTOR	259.59	2.60	263.59	2.93	229.97	**2.55**	231.58	2.57
COUMADIN 5MG (warfarin sodium 5mg)	16.27	**.16**	39.99	.39	34.99	.39	48.15	.48
DEPAKOTE 250MG EC	120.47	1.20	134.99	1.35	72.53	1.21	74.00	**.74**
DETROL LA 4MG SA	300.27	3.00	257.99	2.87	245.97	**2.73**	N/A	N/A
DIFLUCAN 150MG	399.47	**13.32**	64.39	21.46	61.58	15.40	109.78	21.96
DILANTIN 100MG cap. (phenytoin sodium) ES	30.49	.30	35.99	.35	30.40	.34	23.78	**.23**

Drug								
Diltiazem hcl 240mg cap sa	.56	56.39	1.42	127.59	N/A	N/A	187.37	1.89
EFFEXOR XR 75MG cap sa	3.04	303.97	3.62	216.99	259.97	2.89	207.77	2.08
Enalapril maleate 10mg	.14	13.59	.62	36.99	16.99	.18	19.02	.19
Estradiol 2 mg.	.14	13.59	.48	28.99	16.43	.18	17.91	.17
EVISTA 60MG	2.69	269.37	2.66	238.59	222.97	2.47	191.37	2.28
Famotidine 40mg	N/A	N/A	.58	57.99	N/A	N/A	550.49	.56
FLONASE	60.46	181.29	65.63	196.89	179.97	59.99	43.61	.44
Fluoxetine 20mg cap	.13	13.32	.60	53.89	29.97	.33	138.72	1.39
FOSAMAX 10MG	2.43	242.99	2.70	42.89	207.97	2.31	82.80	2.76
Furosemide 40mg	.07	7.49	.12	11.99	8.99	.09	17.12	.17
Gemfibrozil 600mg	.32	32.39	.17	10.39	16.99	.28	29.37	.50
Glipizide er 10mg	.16	15.79	.32	32.99	10.99	.18	20.76	.21
GLUCOPHAGE XR 500MG SA (metformin hcl)	.81	80.89	.92	92.99	47.99	.83	29.92	.29
GLUCOTROL XL 10MG SA (glipizide er 10mg)	.89	89.17	1.17	117.99	68.99	.78	N/A	N/A
IMITREX 50MG	16.83	454.29	18.66	503.89	415.97	15.41	45.25	11.31
K-DUR 20MEQ SA (klor-con M20)	.64	64.69	N/a	N/A	62.23	.62	43.01	.43
LASIX 40MG (furosemide)	.24	23.99	.36	36.99	N/A	N/A	32.17	.36
LEVITRA 10MG	8.69	68.97	10.40	311.89	253.97	8.47	N/A	N/A
LEVOXIL 100 mcg	.28	28.29	.47	46.99	24.97	.28	N/A	N/A
LIPITOR 10MG	2.32	232.07	2.28	205.29	187.97	2.09	95.69	2.13
LIPITOR 20MG	3.22	322.27	3.39	305.19	275.97	3.07	117.25	2.61
Lisinopril HCTZ 10mg	.14	14.49	.49	29.59	47.99	.53	83.74	.84
LOPRESSOR 50MG	1.04	104.19	1.22	72.99	N/A	N/A	42.71	.42
LEXAPRO 20MG	2.28	228.39	2.37	213.59	182.97	2.03	64.21	2.14
LOTENSIN 20MG	1.12	112.39	1.28	76.99	N/A	N/A	127.14	1.51
Lovastatin 20mg	.60	29.79	.86	77.59	99.99	1.11	138.68	1.39
MERIDIA 10MG	3.12	311.99	3.50	314.89	165.97	2.77	N/A	N/A
Metformin hcl 500mg	.14	14.99	.33	29.99	33.99	.57	19.94	.20
Metoprolol 50mg	.13	12.59	.30	17.99	9.99	.17	17.67	.17
MEVACOR 20MG	2.20	220.59	2.30	206.99	197.98	2.20	235.54	2.61
NASONEX (3)	67.23	201.69	78.96	236.89	181.99	60.66	38.83	38.83
NEXIUM 20MG	4.16	415.77	4.38	393.99	363.97	4.04	80.56	2.88
Nifedipine 20mg	.53	52.99	.30	29.99	121.18	1.35	N/A	N/A
NORVASC 5MG	1.44	143.97	1.42	127.59	123.97	1.38	80.16	1.60
Omeprazole 20mg capsule dr	1.18	118.09	1.31	118.09	93.99	3.13	V/A	N/A
ORTHO EVRA PATCHES-9	12.14	109.29	15.65	140.89	104.99	11.67	25.75	8.58
ORTHO TRI-CYCLEN	36.56	109.69	41.96	125.89	108.97	36.32	21.67	21.67

Paroxetine hcl 20mg	68.69	.68	133.09	1.47	201.97	2.24	130.56	1.45
PAXIL 20MG (paroxetine)	274.69	2.75	246.89	2.75	223.97	2.49	230.31	2.30
PEPCID 20MG(famotidine)	174.67	1.74	N/A	N/A	N/A	N/A	133.90	1.49
PLAVIX 75MG	382.17	3.82	338.49	3.76	329.97	3.67	87.34	3.12
PRAVACHOL 40MG	419.27	4.19	396.79	4.41	349.97	3.89	83.73	2.79
PREMARIN .625MG	96.07	.96	109.99	1.16	83.97	.93	33.75	.34
PREMPRO 0.3-1.5 mg	N/A	N/A	141.39	47.13	99.99	33.33	N/A/	N/A
PREVACID 30MG cap	404.67	4.05	357.79	3.98	361.97	4.02	77.17	2.57
PRILOSEC 20MG DR (omeprazole)	385.19	3.85	374.89	4.17	335.99	3.73	N/A	N/A
PROPECIA	144.17	1.60	155.29	1.73	141.97	1.58	183.19	2.18
PROSCAR 5MG	267.37	2.67	251.99	2.87	219.97	2.44	70.93	2.36
PROZAC 10MG	356.49	3.56	365.89	4.06	122.17	4.07	N/A	N/A
RENOVA .05 cream 40 gm	265.57	88.52	287.89	95.96	101.59	101.59	N/A	N/A
RETIN-A .10 cream 45 gm	313.37	104.46	362.89	120.96	306.13	102.04	N/A	N/A
SINGULAIR 10MG	295.89	2.96	289.99	3.22	N/A	N/A	245.31	2.72
STRATTERA 25MG	304.09	3.04	153.99	3.42	83.99	2.80	N/A	N/A
SYNTHROID 100mcg	48.69	.49	49.99	.50	35.97	.40	25.12	.25
Terazosin 5mg capsule	18.09	.18	85.99	.86	33.99	.38	83.08	.83
Tramadol hcl 50mg	17.01	.17	39.99	.67	51.97	.52	N/A	N/A
ULTRAM 50MG (tramadol hcl 50mg)	116.37	1.16	94.99	.95	74.99	1.25	N/A	N/A
VASOTEC 10MG (enalapril maleate)	55.07	1.10	70.99	1.18	97.99	1.09	136.06	1.51
Warfarin sodium 5mg	16.27	.16	39.99	.40	34.99	.35	38.09	.38
WELLBUTRIN 75MG	116.59	1.17	148.99	1.49	102.17	1.14	N/A	N/A
WELLBUTRIN SR 150MG	101.19	1.69	138.99	2.32	322.97	1.79	71.78	1.20
XENICAL	141.57	1.42	48.77	1.63	139.99	1.56	172.44	2.05
ZOCOR 20MG	414.19	4.14	131.99	4.40	356.97	3.97	93.80	3.13
ZOLOFT 50MG	248.37	2.48	85.99	2.87	209.97	3.33	215.54	2.16
ZYBAN	229.87	1.92	SR 142.99	2.37	338.31	1.88	84.94	1.42
ZYPREXA 2.5MG	574.39	5.74	548.89	6.09	431.97	4.79	209.67	2.09
ZYRTEC 10MG	196.99	1.97	183.09	2.03	162.99	1.91	90.74	.90

PLEASE NOTE: PRICES ARE SUBJECT TO CHANGE AND ARE BASED ON RESEARCH IN APRIL 2005. AS A MEMBER, PLEASE LOG ON TO www.prescriptionpathway.com. FOR PRICES THAT ARE UPDATED MONTHLY.

APPENDIX B

APPENDIX B
50 Common Generic Drugs & Brand Name Equivalents

Generic Name	Common Brand Name
1. Hydrocodone with acetaminophen	Vicodin
2. Atenolol	Tenormin
3. Lisinopril	Prinivil or Zestril
4. Albuterol	Proventil or Ventolin
5. Alprazolam	Xanax
6. Hydrochlorathiazide	Microzide
7. Metformin HCL	Glucophage
8. Levothyroxine Sodium	Synthroid
9. Amoxicillin	Amoxil
10. Cephalexin	Keflex
11. Furosemide	Lasix
12. Fluoxetine HCL	Prozac
13. Prednisone	Deltasone
14. Propoxyphene	Darvon
15. Paroxetine	Paxil
16. Triamterene W/HCTZ	Dyazide
17. Omeprazole	Prilosec
18. Metoprolol Tartrate	Lopressor
19. Amitriptyline HCL	Elavil
20. Cyclobenzaprine HCL	Flexeril
21. Lorazepam	Ativan
22. Ranitidine HCL	Zantac
23. Cimetidine	Tagamet
24. Clonoazepam	Klonopin
25. Promethazine HCL	Phenergan
26. Acetaminophen W/Codeine	Tylenol #3 & #4

	Generic Name	Common Brand Name
27.	Medroxyprogesterone Acetate Injectable	Depo-Provera
28.	Verapamil HCL	Isoptin
29.	Estradiol	Estrace
30.	Lovastatin	Mevacor
31.	Loratadine	Claritin
32.	Trazodone HCL	Desyrel
33.	Doxazosin Mesylate	Cardura
34.	Phenytoin	Dilantin
35.	Diazepam	Valium
36.	Allopurinol	Zyloprim
37.	Acyclovir	Zovirax
38.	Warfarin Sodium	Coumadin
39.	Glyburide	Micronase
40.	Minocycline HCL	Minocin
41.	Gemfibrozil	Lopid
42.	Oxycodone w/Acetominophen	Percocet
43.	Promethazine HCL	Phenergan
44.	Doxycycline Hyclate	Vibramycin
45.	Methylprednisolone	Medrol
46.	Fluconazole	Diflucan
47.	Naproxyn	Naprosyn
48.	Carisoprodol	Soma
49.	Nitroglycerin	Nitrodur
50.	Metronidazole	Flagyl

APPENDIX C

APPENDIX C

Personal Medication Record
Checkbook Size

Take the form on the following page to the physician's office for an "Rx Tune-up"- then every office visit thereafter.

Date began taking	Prescription drug name	Dosage	How much to take and when (e.g. 1 - 4 x a day)	Do not take with (antacids, grapefruit)
	OTC drug name			
	Vitamins & Nutritional Supplements Name			

3 Questions to ask your Physician and Pharmacist _each_ time a new prescription drug is purchased:

Name: Address: Phone #:	Drug Allergies: Emergency Contact:	
1. Is this a generic? If not, why not?		
2. Do I have any diseases or conditions that would keep me from taking this drug?		
3. Will this drug interact with any OTC drugs, vitamins, or nutritional supplements I am taking?		

APPENDIX D

APPENDIX D

COST SAVINGS WORKSHEET

NAME OF DRUG	YOUR PRICE/YR.	NEW PRICE /YR.	YOU SAVE
OTCs			
Dietary Supplements			
Total $:			
Comparison Shopping Saves You: Annual Percentage Savings:			$ ____ ____ %

APPENDIX E

IMPORTANT NOTICE

Prescription Pathway website

Access the www.prescriptionpathway.com website for current information:

In order to review prescription drug updates and to receive a free bimonthly newsletter, readers can log on to: www.prescriptionpathway.com. Click "members LogIn" Under user id, enter: prescriptionpathway. When you are prompted to enter the password, enter: discounts

REFERENCES

Introduction
1. U.S. Bureau of Labor Statistics, Consumer Expenditure Survey. 2000.
2. National Association of Chain Drug Stores, NACD, manufacturer sales data from IMS Health used with the addition of a retail margin to estimate retail sales. Available at http://www.macds.org/wmsprint/cfm?print_url=http%3A/www.nacds.org/wmspage.cfm%. Accessed June 10, 2005.
3. AP/Ipsos Poll:" Americans Mostly Confident Prescription Drugs are Safe." Ipsos-Public Affairs December 21, 2004.

Chapter 1
1. Center for Medicare & Medicare Services. Health Care Industry Market Update. January 2003.
2. National Association of Chain Drug Stores, NACD, manufacturer sales data from IMS Health used with the addition of a retail margin to estimate retail sales. Available at http://www.macds.org/wmsprint/cfm?print_url=http%3A/www.nacds.org/wmspage.cfm%. Accessed June 10, 2005.
3. IMS Health Inc. "Retail Prescription Growth at Record Level in 2003." Available at http:www.imshealthcanada.com/htmen/4_2_1_49.htm. Accessed December 6, 2004.
4. CDC. "Physician Visits Reach 824 Million in 2000." Available at http://www.cdc.gov/nchs/releases/02news/physician.htm. Accessed March 5, 2003.
5. Kaiser Family Foundation. "Prescription Drug Trends". Source: IMS Health. Available at http://www.kff.org. Accessed March 2003.
6. National Association of Chain Drug Stores, NACD, manufacturer sales data from IMS Health used with the addition of a retail margin to estimate retail sales. Available at http://www.macds.org/wmsprint/cfm?print_url=http%3A/www.nacds.org/wmspage.cfm%. Accessed June 10, 2005.
7. The National Institute for Health Care Management Research and Education Foundation. "Prescription Drug Expenditures in 2001: Another Year of Escalating Costs". April 2002; 6-8. Available at http://www.nihcm.org. Accessed January 2003.
8. CDC. "National Ambulatory Medical Care Survey: 2000 Summary". June 5, 2002; Number 328:7. Available at http://www.cdc.gov.
9. Monster.com. Pharmacy Feature: "Natural, Not Necessarily Safe." Available at http://content.myh.monster.com/pharmacy features. asp. Accessed June 3, 2002.
10. Ballington, Don A., Laughlin, Mary M., Pharmacology for Technicians, Paradigm Publishing, 1999, p. 3.

11. Ibid, p. 4.
12. IMS Health Inc. IMS Retail Drug Monitor Hot Topics.June2003.
13. Beer, Mark H. M.D. Merck Manual of Medical Information. Second Home Addition. Pocket Books, division of Simon and Schuster, 2003. p.60.
14. IBID
15. National Association of Chain Drug Stores, NACD, manufacturer sales data from IMS Health used with the addition of a retail margin to estimate retail sales. Available at http://www.macds.org/wmsprint/cfm?print_url=http%3A/www.nacds.org/wmspage.cfm%. Accessed June 10, 2005.

Chapter 2

1. IMS Health. "Pharmaceutical Market Intelligence". Available at http://www.open.imshealth.com/IMSinclude/i_article_20040623a.asp. Accessed July 2, 20004.
2. IBID
3. Food & Drug Administration. "Science Meets Beauty: Using Medicine to Improve Appearances." Available at http://www.fda.gov/fdac/features/2004/204_beauty.html). Accessed November 26, 2004.
4. IMS Health. "IMS highlights biotech as strong growth driver." June 23, 2004. Available at http://www.open.imshealth.com/IMSinclude/i_article_20040623.asp. Accessed July 2, 2004.
5. Clinical trials.com. Frequently Asked Questions. Available at http://www.clinicaltrials.com/FAQ/faq.asp. Accessed June 6, 2004.
6. FDAnews Drug Bulletin™. Vol.2, No.50. 3/11/05.
7. Hawthorne, Fran. The Merck Druggernaut. John Wiley & Sons, Inc. 2003. pp. 66-67
8. Barlett, Donald L., and Steele, James B., "Why We Pay So Much For Drugs," TIME February 2, 2004.
9. Hawthorne, Fran. The Merck Druggernaut. John Wiley & Sons, Inc. 2003. p.109.
10. Marsa, Linda. "Medical Marvels". America West. May 2003.
11. Hawthorne, Fran. The Merck Druggernaut. John Wiley & Sons, Inc. 2003. p. 179
12. Marsa, Linda. Medical Marvels. America West. May 2003.
13. IBID
14. Centerwatch.com. Available at http://www.centerwatch.com/patient/backgrnd.html. Accessed 6/12/04.

Chapter 3

1. "It's a Wonderful Life." Produced and directed by Frank Capra. RKO studios, 1946.

2. AP/Ipsos Poll:" Americans Mostly Confident Prescription Drugs are Safe." Ipsos-Public Affairs December 21, 2004.
3. FDAnews Drug Bulletin™. Vol.1, No.122. 7/2/04.
4. Food and Drug Administration. "FDA tips for taking medicines from FDA Consumer." FDA Consumer. August 01.
5. AHRQ & NCPIE. "Your Medicine: Play it safe." Available at www.ahrq.gov/consumer/safemeds/safemeds.htm. Accessed 5/7/03.
6. Johnson, Lane P., MD. MPH, "Pocket Guide to Herbal Remedies." Blackwell Science Inc. 2002. p.xvii.
7. Wolfe, Sidney, M.D, Sasich, Larry, PharmD, MPH, Hayes, Rose Ellen, RPh, and Public Citizen's Health Research Group, "Worst Pills, Best Pills," Pocket Books. 1999. p.17.
8. Appleby, Julie, "Fake drugs show up in U.S. pharmacies as prescription prices rise, counterfeiters chase profits." USA TODAY. Available at http://www.usatoday.com/usaonline/20030515/5159798s.htm. Accessed 6/19/03.
9. Appleby, Julie, "Blister packs could be weapon to fight fake drugs." USA TODAY.
10. Eban, Katherine "It's a FAKE and your pharmacist doesn't know it," Self magazine. 2003.

Chapter 4

1. Managed Care Institute, Samford University. September 2000.
2. Barr Labs. Available at http://www.barrlabs.com/pages/faqcon.htm. Accessed 11/26/04.
3. IBID
4. Food & Drug Administration. Available at www.fda.gov/cder/consumerinfo/generic_equivalence.htm. Accessed 11/26/04.
5. Abboud, Leila and Mathews, Anna Wilde, The Wall Street Journal, Oct. 14, 2003.
6. "Annual Drug Trend Report" Medco. 2004.
7. Consumer Reports. 2005 Guide to Diet, Health & Fitness. Shoreline Publishing Group LLC. 2005.
8. "Side Effects of New Drugs Often Take Time to Arise, Study Says." The Wall Street Journal. May 1, 2002.

Chapter 5

1. Barlett, Donald L., and Steele, James B., "Why We Pay So Much For Drugs", TIME February 2, 2004.
2. Kaiser Family Foundation. "Trends and Indicators in the Changing Health Care Marketplace". Available at http://www.kff.org/insurance/7031/ti2004-1-21.cfm. Accessed 6/19/05

3. IMS Health. "Generics Flourish as Innovation Stalls". June 23, 2004. Available at http://www.www.open.imshealth.com/IMSinclude/i_article_20040623a.asp

4. HarrisInteractive. "Reputations of Pharmaceutical and Health Insurance Continue their Downward Slide." Available at http://www.harrisinteractive.com/news/allnewsbydate.asp?NewsID=814. Accessed on 6/19/05.

5. Welch, William M. "Drug prices outstrip inflation." USA TODAY. Available at http://www.usatoday.com. Accessed 6/19/05

6. Hawthorne, Fran. The Merck Druggernaut. John Wiley & Sons, Inc. 2003. p.166.

7. "Pharmaceutical Industry profile 2005. PhRMA. Available at http://www.phrma.org

8. Drinkard, Jim. "Drugmakers go furthest to sway Congress: USA TODAY. 4/26/05

9. Hawthorne, Fran. The Merck Druggernaut. John Wiley & Sons, Inc. 2003. p.181.

10. Goozner, Merrill "The $800 Million Pill." University of California. 2004.

11. "The Off-Label Crisis Workshop". Available at http://www.products@enewsletters.fdanews.com Accessed 2/18/05.

12. Hawthorne, Fran. The Merck Druggernaut. John Wiley & Sons, Inc. 2003. p.133.

13. IBID p.142.

14. Szabo, Liz. "Health systems cutting costs by closing door on drug reps". USA TODAY. 8/25/04.

15. IBID.

16. Hawthorne, Fran. The Merck Druggernaut. John Wiley & Sons, Inc. 2003. p.196.

17. Readers Digest. October 2003.

18. Schmidt, Julie. "Drugmakers likely to lob softer pitches" USA TODAY. 3/11/05.

19. Mack, John. "The Targeted Model: The Future of Pharmaceutical Marketing?" VirSci Corp. www.virsci.com. July/August 2004.

20. Hawthorne, Fran. The Merck Druggernaut. John Wiley & Sons, Inc. 2003. p.17, p.244.

21. MacKinnon, Neil J. "Use of drug samples as a threat to seamless health care" AM J Health-Syst Pharm. 2004:61:1497-500.

22. National Consumer League. Available at http://www.NCLnet.org/thesurvey. February 2003.

23. Manning, Anita. "Plugged into prescription drugs." USA TODAY. 2/15/05.

24. IBID. USA TODAY reports from an article appearing in The New England Journal of Medicine.

25. Appleby, Julie. "Web site compares drugs for 'best buys'". USA TODAY. 12/9/04.

Chapter 6

1. Appleby, Julie. "HMO premiums expected to increase yet again." USA TODAY. 6/10/05.
2. IMS Health. As quoted from the FDAnews Drug Daily Bulletin. Vol.1. No.20 2/6/04.
3. Pallarito, Karen. "Consumers Seen as Key to Controlling Health Costs." REUTERS. 3/14/03.
4. Bootman, J. Lyle, PhD. "The Need to Understand Cost & Quality: A Case for Chronic Care". 6/18/05
5. Freudenheim, Milt. "Drugstores Fret as Insurers Demand Pills by Mail". New York Times. 1/1/05.
6. Kaiser Family Foundation. "Follow the Pill: Understanding the U.S. Commercial Pharmaceutical Supply Chain." Prepared for KFF by the Health Strategies Consultancy, LLC. March 2005. Available at http:/www.kff.org.
7. Szabo, Liz. "Health systems cutting costs by closing door on drug reps". USA TODAY. 8/25/04
8. U.S. DHHS. Agency for Healthcare Research and Quality. "Significant increases in drug copayments may reduce patients' use of needed medications." AHRQ Research Activities. No. 285, May 2004.
9. Drs. Jason Theodosakis, & David T. Feinberg. "When Your Insurance Won't Pay. Parade. September 19, 2004.

Chapter 7

1. Thomas, Cindy Parks, PhD., et. al. "PBM-Administered Prescription Drug Discount Cards." Prepared by Brandeis University Schneider Institute for Health Policy. Available at http://www.heller.brandeis.edu/welcome/news research.asp?ResearchNumber=1. 9/11/04.
2. United States General Accounting Office. "Prescription Drug Discount Cards. Savings Depend on Pharmacy and Type of Card Used." September 2003.

Chapter 8

1. Monica Mathys, Pharm.D, CGP, Presentation: "Tips for Determining Appropriate Drug Therapy in the Elderly" at the APA Meeting, June 25, 2004.
2. Pear, Robert, "Lottery Planned for Test of Medicare's New Drug Coverage." The New York Times. 6/2504. Available at nytimes.com.
3. Reuters. "Focus groups: Medicare drug plan confusing". Available at cnn.com. 6/4/04.
4. Henry J. Kaiser Family Foundation, Medicare- Medicare+Choice Fact Sheet #2052-06. April 2003.
5. Freudenheim, Milt. "Using New Medicare Billions, H.M.O.s Again Court Elderly" The New York Times. 3/9/04.

6.   Monica Mathys, Pharm.D, CGP, Presentation: "Tips for Determining Appropriate Drug Therapy in the Elderly" at the APA Meeting, June 26, 2004.
7.   U.S. DHHS. Agency for Healthcare Research and Quality. "Potentially inappropriate medications are prescribed for up to one in five elderly people." AHRQ Research Activities. No. 285, May 2004.
8.   U.S. General Accounting Office. Available at USP Patient Safety CAPSLink Newsletter. November 2003.
9.   Henry J. Kaiser Family Foundation, Medicare- Medicare+Choice Fact Sheet #2052-06. April 2003.

Chapter 9

1.   "Paying the Price: A 19-State Survey of the High Cost of Prescription Drugs." National Assoc. of State Public Interest Research Group. July 2003

Chapter 10

1.   Covington, Tim R., M.S. Pharm D. "Rx to OTC Switches: Opportunity for Pharmacy". Presentation at APA Meeting. June 26, 2004.
2.   IBID
3.   IBID
4.   NCPIE. "Uses and Attitudes About Taking Over-the-Counter Medicines": National Council on Patient Information and Education (NCPIE). Accessed at http://www.bemedwise.org 11/2/04
5.   APHA. "What you should know abut Over-the-Counter Medicines and Drug Interactions." American Pharmacists Association. December 2003.
6.   "The purple pill heads over-the-counter." Available at http:www/cnn.com. Accessed 9/18/03.

Chapter 11

1.   "Aisles of Opportunity". MM& M. October, 2004
2.   2005 Guide to Diet, Health & Fitness. Consumer Reports. Time Inc. Home Entertainment. 2005.
3.   Freudenheim, Milt. "Drugstores Fret as Insurers Demand Pills by Mail". New York Times. 1/1/05.
4.   "What is Pill-Splitting"? Available at http://www.OregonRx.org/gov/DAS/OHPPR/ORRX/pt_pill_splitting.shtml. Accessed 12/8/04.

Chapter 12

1.   Forrester Research. "Survey: Few Consumers Buy Medications Online." Available at http://www.ihealthbeat.org/index.cfm. January 2005. Accessed 2/3/05.
2.   IBID

3.   ITFacts based on JupiterResearch. Available at
      http://www.itfacts.biz/index.php?id=P1307. Accessed 11/24/04.
4.   IBID

Chapter 13
1.   Barlett, Donald L., and Steele, James B., "Why We Pay So Much For Drugs",
      TIME February 2, 2004.
2.   IBID
3.   IBID

Chapter 14
1.   Goldberg, Robert, M.D. "Does Importation Save Money and Lives?
      Not in Europe." Medical Progress Today. September 29, 2004.
2.   "Pfizer, Canadian Pharmacies Take Drug Fight to Europe." Available at
      http://www.bloomberg.com. Accessed 5/17/05.
3.   IBID
4.   "Illinois to Buy Drugs in Australia, New Zealand, Governor Says." Available
      at http://www.bloomberg.com. Accessed on 7/19/05.

Chapter 15
1.   Wagner, Dennis, U.S. Department of State, Mexican law enforcement
      authorities, Mexican pharmacists and www.drugbuyers.com., as written in
      The Arizona Republic, July 9,2004.

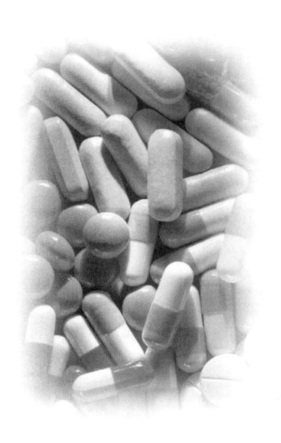